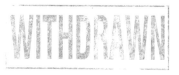
NFUL BLADDER SYNDROME

by the same author

Make Yourself Better
A Practical Guide to Restoring Your Body's
Wellbeing through Ancient Medicine
Philip Weeks
ISBN 978 1 84819 012 2
eISBN 978 0 85701 077 3

of related interest

The Functional Nutrition Cookbook
Addressing Biochemical Imbalances through Diet
Lorraine Nicolle and Christine Bailey
ISBN 978 1 84819 079 5
eISBN 978 0 85701 052 0

Breaking Free from Persistent Fatigue
Lucie Montpetit
ISBN 978 1 84819 101 3
eISBN 978 0 85701 081 0

Managing Stress with Qigong
Gordon Faulkner
Foreword by Carole Bridge
ISBN 978 1 84819 035 1
eISBN 978 0 85701 016 2

PAINFUL BLADDER SYNDROME

CONTROLLING AND RESOLVING
INTERSTITIAL CYSTITIS THROUGH
NATURAL MEDICINE

PHILIP WEEKS

SINGING
DRAGON

LONDON AND PHILADELPHIA

First published in 2013
by Singing Dragon
an imprint of Jessica Kingsley Publishers
116 Pentonville Road
London N1 9JB, UK
and
400 Market Street, Suite 400
Philadelphia, PA 19106, USA

www.singingdragon.com

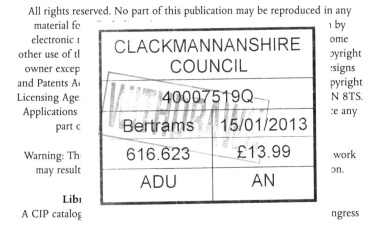

British Library Cataloguing in Publication Data
A CIP catalogue record for this book is available from the British Library

ISBN 978 1 84819 110 5
eISBN 978 0 85701 089 6

Printed and bound in Great Britain

Contents

Disclaimer

If you decide to make any lifestyle changes or undertake a cleanse/detox routine, you will first need to consult a medical doctor and/or a suitably qualified practitioner. They will assess whether any of the changes or routines are suitable for you by considering your current state of health and pre-existing conditions, as well as any medication you may be taking or have taken in the past.

Many foods, herbs and spices can occasionally cause allergic reactions. Any of the recommendations in this book could be potentially dangerous, even deadly, especially if you are already ill or suffer from a disease.

Every effort has been made to ensure that the information contained in this book is correct, but it should not in any way be substituted for medical advice. Readers should always consult a qualified medical practitioner before incorporating any of the therapies mentioned in this book into their treatment plan, whether conventional, complementary or alternative. Neither the author nor the publisher take any responsibility for the consequences of any decision made as a result of the information contained in this book.

Introduction

The seeds for this book were sown some 12 years ago. A woman in her mid-40s who had been suffering from almost a year of horrendous bladder pain and an unrelenting feeling of burning and irritation when urinating consulted me. Before seeing me she had all of the standard medical tests offered to her, which had come back clear; she was discharged, with painkillers and antibiotics.

From my analysis, I discovered a number of imbalances. Although in theory they were straightforward, careful attention would be needed to address them. Before the bladder pain had manifested, she had experienced an almost constant urinary tract infection for 18 months. Antibiotics would clear it up, and then it would come back. This cycle had been continuing every few weeks.

When I first saw her, she was experiencing bouts of thrush, as well as symptoms of irritable bowel syndrome (IBS) and frequent headaches.

Because the antibiotics she was prescribed are fairly indiscriminate with the bacteria they kill, she was severely lacking in the beneficial bacteria in her digestive system. This was leading to her body not being able to control fungus, and she had serious yeast overgrowth. Typically in this situation, not only is the gut suffering, so that she is struggling to digest her food properly, but also the immune system is struggling to control inflammation.

A routine of taking beneficial bacteria, antifungals and herbal teas for her bladder had a remarkable effect and she became free of pain and symptoms. Since that time I have seen many people improve who were once in a bleak cycle of pain and despair.

I certainly wouldn't say I have the only solution and final word to say about painful bladder syndrome (PBS) (also known as interstitial cystitis, which is abbreviated to IC). Through working with this disorder I haven't found one single isolated cause or solution; however, I have treated people who have recovered and become symptom-free.

The people who come to see me tend to have already tried the orthodox approach and, for whatever reason, it is no longer working for them.

My interest with any health condition is why is the body not healing itself? In my first book, *Make Yourself Better*, I explore the key factors I see in my clinical practice which are influencing people's 'level of health'. Although orthodox medical approaches have provided immense solutions for many of the health problems that were once life threatening, the new plagues are chronic, often unresponsive to orthodox treatments and are having a profound negative effect on our lives and wellbeing.

In this book I cover the key areas that I believe should be addressed if you want to support your body with PBS. I am not claiming I have a cure, because I don't. I also believe that orthodox medicine has a very important role to play. However, I have seen extraordinary changes occur in people's health once the blocks to healing have been resolved. This usually means stopping the things that are contributing to the problem, often foods and lifestyle habits, and giving the body what it needs to repair itself.

I discuss dietary factors, which means not just avoiding foods that aggravate your system, but eating foods which are important in repairing the bladder lining itself.

Herbs are an incredibly important part of my programme, and I discuss my formulas that I have found useful in my clinical practice.

Increasingly I find that our bodies are overburdened with toxins from our modern world. And although it is essential for these to be released from the body, it needs to be done in a way which doesn't exacerbate the problem. Invariably I find that health crises have a trigger, often through events in our lives, some kind of shock or stress. This affects our underlying health and the capacity to repair. I discuss ways that the effects of trauma and stress can be released and how we can take steps to restore our capacity to heal.

Flare-ups can always be a potential and I discuss ways that these can be tackled as well as preventing and treating urinary tract infections.

If you have PBS, then what I can say is that there is a way. There will be a personal solution for you to repair, heal and get well again.

PART I

Understanding Painful Bladder Syndrome

CHAPTER 1

What is Painful Bladder Syndrome?

The short answer is that painful bladder syndrome is a chronic condition in which the bladder wall becomes inflamed, causing bladder pain, urinary urgency and increased frequency. However, as 70 per cent of people with painful bladder syndrome also have coexisting and related conditions, they can experience several other symptoms besides. It is widely considered that 'painful bladder syndrome is a disease which profoundly affects patients' quality of life due to disabling symptoms.'[1]

A protective layer made up of glycosaminoglycans – or GAGs – which is a component of the bladder wall protects the bladder from the harmful substances in our urine. In painful bladder syndrome/interstitial cystitis (IC) this protecting layer is thought to be thinner,[2,3] making it defective, thus exposing the bladder wall to the impurities contained in urine, which in turn causes inflammation and pain.

Unlike the more commonly occurring forms of cystitis, a urine sample from someone with painful bladder syndrome rarely reveals an active infection; the symptoms experienced by patients are believed to be due to damage or injury to the bladder lining. This means that it won't respond to antibiotics that would ordinarily work with bacterial cystitis.

It also means that symptoms can last far longer, though some patients can have periods of remission.

In the UK alone, some 400,000 people are estimated to have painful bladder syndrome, with women making up 90 per cent of that figure.[4] It can affect people of any age, even children.

Compared with other diseases, very little is known or proven about painful bladder syndrome. Its causes are yet to be fully established – though defective bladder lining is a key suspect – and diagnosis is fraught with difficulty. Painful bladder syndrome can evade clinical detection procedures such as scans and urine cytology tests and, in any case, its symptoms are very similar to those of many other diseases. So, where a person is experiencing bladder pain, frequency and urgency, diagnosis of painful bladder syndrome is usually established by ruling out those other diseases.

The term bladder pain syndrome evolved when it became apparent that many people's experience did not reflect the exact scientific definition of the more commonly occurring cystitis. Examples are patients who do not have Hunner's ulcers or glomerulations in the bladder, or who are able to sleep through the night without waking regularly to urinate.

During your research into painful bladder syndrome, you will probably also come across the terms interstitial cystitis, hypersensitive bladder syndrome, bladder pain syndrome, IC and PBS. All these are alternative names for painful bladder syndrome, which from this point on I shall refer to simply as PBS.

It is beyond the scope of this book to delve too deeply into what can and cannot be proven about PBS. Nor do I wish to blind you with too much science or medical jargon – although some terminology is impossible to avoid. What I have set out to do is to help you understand what we do know about PBS and how you can develop a strategy to meet it head on – and minimise its impact on your life.

Symptoms of PBS

As mentioned above, there are three main symptoms associated with PBS – pain, urgency and frequency. Women may experience pain in the abdomen, urethra and vaginal area, particularly during lovemaking, while men can feel pain in the testicles, scrotum and perineum and experience discomfort when ejaculating. Urgency is the feeling of being 'caught short' – the immediate need to urinate – sometimes causing pain, pressure or spasm, while frequency refers to a dramatic increase in toilet visits. For some people, this can be as many as 60 times over a 24-hour period. This inevitably includes getting up several times in the night to urinate, a condition known as nocturia.

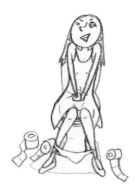

Most people with PBS (90%) have the non-ulcerative form of the disease. In some cases they may have tiny haemorrhages, called glomerulations, on the bladder wall, which usually indicates the ulcerative form of PBS. However, glomerulations are not necessarily proof that a patient has PBS as they can appear with any disorder which inflames the bladder.

The 10 per cent of patients with ulcerative PBS usually also have Hunner's ulcers. These form on the bladder wall, vary in size and can bleed. Though defined as ulcers, they are in fact areas of inflammation. Unlike glomerulations, Hunner's ulcers are specific to PBS and their presence will confirm a positive diagnosis.

In severe cases of PBS, patients can experience its symptoms for more than two years and possibly develop what is known as End Stage PBS. This is where the bladder is very hard, has a low capacity and causes a high level of pain. Around 5 per cent of people with PBS have it in this form.

I want to emphasise that, for some, the distress caused by PBS can be immense. Many of the people I have come into contact with who have the condition have found it so unbearable that they have contemplated suicide. I often hear stories involving years of misdiagnosis and uncertainty.

The difficulty with PBS is that there isn't an absolute and definitive test which can determine whether someone has it or not. Those who have ulcers on the bladder can be told with certainty that they have the condition, but many people have all of the symptoms without any evidence of ulcerations and PBS is diagnosed only because all other lines of enquiry have been exhausted. This can be incredibly frustrating for patients and physicians alike.

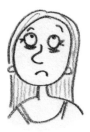

The kidneys

Let's have a quick look at the kidneys and bladder so we can visualise what is going on in the body. Sited either side of the spine at the back of the abdomen, the kidneys are involved in several functions vital to our health. While central to the urinary system they also regulate electrolytes and help to maintain the balance of salt and water in the body, and thereby our acid balance. Other functions of the kidneys include reabsorbing amino acids, water and glucose and producing hormones and enzymes.

Blood entering the kidneys through the renal arteries gets drained into the renal veins. The kidneys then filter the blood, removing the waste products, urea and ammonium. The kidneys then produce urine, which carries these waste products to the bladder through little tubes called ureters, ready for excreting out of the body.

Due to the shape of the liver, the position of the kidneys is not symmetrical. The right kidney sits slightly lower and more off centre than its left counterpart and is also slightly smaller. A typical kidney is 11–14cm long, around 6cm wide and 4cm thick. Weight varies from around 125 to 170 grams in adult men and a fractionally lighter 115 to 155 grams in adult women.

The kidneys, and the adrenal glands which sit on top of them, are protected by a tough tissue known as the renal capsule, a double layer of fat and a further layer of connective tissue known as the renal fascia.

The parts of the kidneys responsible for producing urine are known as nephrons. These span both the deep (medulla) and the superficial (cortex) structures of the kidney. Through a complex system of ducts, the nephrons draw waste products into the urine and drain it into a collection duct. From here, the urine passes through organs called calyces before being emptied into the ureters for its onward passage to the bladder.

Due to its close relationship with the bladder and the influence it has in the toxicity of urine, I believe maintaining good kidney health through diet and regular detoxification plays a major role in managing PBS symptoms.

The bladder

After leaving the kidneys and passing through the ureters, urine arrives in the bladder where it is stored prior to urination. The bladder is located upon the pelvic floor. In men it sits between the rectum at the rear and the joint that connects the two halves of the pelvis (pubic symphysis) at the front. Beneath the male bladder is the prostate. The female bladder is slightly smaller and sits in front of the vagina, beneath the uterus. Both the male and female bladders excrete urine from the body through the urethra.

The bladder is a muscular hollow, elastic organ that expands as it fills with urine. As it does so, the bladder wall becomes thinner in order to minimise the pressure we experience. When the bladder is stretched to its maximum, a muscle known as the detrusor, which forms part of the bladder wall, contracts to expel the urine into the urethra.

The male urethra, which travels through the penis and also delivers semen during climax, is longer than the female urethra which carries only urine and terminates above the opening of the vagina. The male urethra also differs from the female organ in that it is formed of four parts:

- *Pre-prostatic urethra*: the section between the bladder and the prostate gland, measuring approximately 0.5– 1.5cm depending on bladder fullness.

- *Prostatic urethra*: the section that passes through the prostate gland. Here the urethra has openings called verumontanum to receive sperm and seminal fluids.

- *Membranous urethra*: a 1–2cm section that passes through the external urethral sphincter.

- *Spongy urethra*: the final length of the urethra running the length of the penis. The internal structure of this section creates a spiral stream of urine which has a cleansing effect. This is understood to be one of the reasons why urinary tract infections (UTIs) occur less frequently in men than in women. On the other hand, the male urethra features a prominent bend, which makes catheterisation more complicated for men than for women.

In both sexes, the involuntary flow of urine is controlled by the urethral sphincter. This is the muscle we contract when 'holding it in'.

CHAPTER 2

Diagnosing Painful Bladder Syndrome

Because it shares several symptoms with other conditions, many of which may also be present in patients, diagnosing PBS is notoriously difficult. Patients are often misdiagnosed and treated for overactive bladder, haemorrhagic cystitis, urinary tract infections (UTIs) or, in the case of many men, chronic prostatitis/chronic pelvic pain syndrome (CP/CPPS), only to experience the continued discomfort of PBS.

The most important diseases to rule out are urinary tract cancer and bladder cancer. It is only when these and all other diseases are excluded that your doctors can say with any certainty that you have PBS. This involves checking for tenderness and any abnormal growths around your abdomen and pelvic area and testing for inflammations and infections that cause similar symptoms to those of PBS. Urine tests are also commonplace to help rule out UTIs. Your doctors will also discuss the severity of your symptoms with you and devise a regime to manage your pain.

These measures effectively enable a diagnosis of PBS/interstitial cystitis (IC) to be made through a process of elimination. Once your doctors are reasonably sure that you have PBS, they may want to perform a test known as a cystoscopy with hydrodistention which will help to confirm the diagnosis.

Cystoscopy with hydrodistention

Simply put, this involves gently stretching the bladder by filling it with fluid (hydrodistention), then inserting a tiny camera called a cystoscope inside through the urethra to look for clues signalling the presence of PBS on the bladder wall. These include glomerulations, Hunner's ulcers and other abnormalities. The procedure is carried out under local or general anaesthetic and takes no more than 15 minutes.

It's also possible to fit instruments to a cystoscope for obtaining a biopsy of the bladder wall during a cystoscopy. This can help to rule out bladder cancer.

For some patients, hydrodistention has a therapeutic as well as diagnostic benefit, with some reporting the alleviation of pain and discomfort for up to six months. In such cases, patients have made the procedure a regular part of their pain management. Similarly, a cystoscopy can help to break down scar tissue on the wall of the bladder, giving temporary pain relief.

If the results of the cystoscopy with hydrodistention confirm that you have PBS, your doctor will schedule a follow-up appointment to discuss your treatment and symptom-relief options. Although it is a more definitive test to determine whether you do have PBS, it is invasive and isn't without its potential side-effects as some, unfortunately, experience pelvic pain, bleeding and urethral burning for some weeks afterwards and require pain-relieving drugs.

PBS – not to be confused with...

As there is no definitive diagnostic test for PBS, misdiagnosis is not uncommon. It's worth familiarising yourself, then, with the conditions most likely to be mistaken for PBS.

Overactive bladder (OAB)

Urgency – the sudden need to go to the toilet – is the symptom most commonly shared by PBS and OAB patients. However, with OAB the need arises as a result of involuntary contractions of a muscle in the bladder wall, called the detrusor. OAB is a nervous dysfunction and not, as with PBS, to do with the glycosaminoglycan (GAG) layer in the bladder wall. It can often be brought under control through a reduction in caffeine and alcohol intake together with a range of bladder training measures and pelvic floor exercises, such as Kegel.

Kegel exercises involve consciously contracting the muscles that you use when you want to stop urinating. The concept behind these exercises is that contracting these muscles strengthens and tones the muscles of the pelvic floor. The exercises can be useful for urinary incontinence and uterine prolapse, and premature ejaculation in men. However, someone with PBS may find that Kegel exercises actually aggravate their symptoms as they are practising 'tightening' their pelvic floor muscles and often they are already chronically tense.

Haemorrhagic cystitis

This is another disorder in which patients experience pain, frequency, urgency and nocturia, but with added symptoms including urine in the blood, systemic infection and urinary obstruction. Usually caused by cancer therapies such as chemotherapy or radiation, haemorrhagic cystitis normally clears up at the end of the treatment.

Urinary tract infection (UTI)

Although PBS patients often experience similar symptoms to those of UTIs, the underlying causes are quite different. UTIs or bladder infections are characterised by bacteria in the urine. UTIs, unlike PBS, can be treated with antibiotics. That said, people with PBS can – and often do – get UTIs as well.

Chronic prostatitis

For men, PBS and chronic prostatitis/chronic pelvic pain syndrome (CP/CPPS) are very similar in their symptoms. Urgency, frequency, nocturia and pain when urinating are characteristic of both conditions. There are, however, therapies for CP/CPPS so continued symptoms after this kind of treatment could signal PBS.

Tina, age 32

Tina had a series of recurring UTIs over a period of three years. Each time the symptoms arose she was prescribed antibiotics. These worked for a while, then ceased to have any effect. This caused Tina both physical discomfort – in the form of pain, a burning sensation when urinating and increased frequency and urgency – and emotional anxiety and a fear that she had an incurable condition or worse, it was all in her head. Tina consulted a urologist who conducted a multitude of tests, none of which revealed any useful information. Pain medication was prescribed but still there was no improvement.

Distraught, Tina went for a second opinion. After a more in-depth evaluation of her symptoms, circumstances and coexisting conditions, Tina was eventually diagnosed with PBS.

With her symptoms now under control, Tina feels a huge relief that she has a treatable condition. She's glad to be off prescription drugs, too.

PBS flare-ups

PBS flare-ups are episodes when the classic PBS symptoms of pain, frequency and urgency become more noticeable over extended periods. Flare-ups vary from patient to patient, with some reporting only a slight worsening of their symptoms for a few hours while others have recorded periods of several weeks during which their pain, frequency and urgency intensified dramatically.

In Chapter 10, we'll take a look at the many ways to combat, and even pre-empt, PBS flare-ups.

The combined effect of all these symptoms can affect a PBS patient's life far beyond the physical discomfort. Sleep deprivation caused by nocturia can result in severe fatigue, while increased daytime frequency can make routine tasks such as travelling, working and shopping a real challenge. By its very nature, PBS can be a cause of intense distress and embarrassment in social or work environments. The impact on physical intimacy can range from putting a real dampener on someone's sex life to making it impossible due to intense pain and discomfort. Clearly, PBS comes with a social dimension and far-reaching lifestyle implications. The Harvard Medical School's Family Health Guide reiterates this:

> Interstitial cystitis is a chronic inflammation of the bladder that causes people to urinate – sometimes painfully – as often as 40, 50, or 60 times a day. Their quality of life, research suggests, resembles that of a person on kidney dialysis or suffering from chronic cancer pain.[5]

The good news is that there are strategies that you can start today that can help you get your life back on track. We'll explore these in detail in Part II.

PBS v. cystitis

Cystitis differs from PBS in that it is an infection of the bladder and urinary tract as opposed to damage of the bladder wall. Cystitis or urinary tract infections (UTIs) come on suddenly, yet are usually short-lived and respond quite quickly to both antibiotics and natural treatments. The symptoms, however, can be very similar and people with PBS are often misdiagnosed as having regularly recurring UTIs through lack of adequate testing and assumptions based on previous infection.

This can lead to patients repeatedly taking antibiotics over extended periods which, I believe, in turn can leave them more exposed to the potential development of PBS. This is because, over time, antibiotics compromise the beneficial flora in the gut, allowing the growth of fungus and undesirable bacteria to reach unmanageable levels, eventually causing changes in the gut called 'gut permeability syndrome' or 'leaky gut'. And as we will see, I believe gut permeability syndrome to play a huge role in PBS and other chronic health conditions.

In my clinical experience I have also seen many patients, who have previously been correctly diagnosed with UTIs, become overmedicated with antibiotics to the point where they have developed PBS as a result of their treatment. While I fully accept the case for orthodox medicine in many cases of cystitis, I am also glad that there is a growing acceptance and recognition of the role that natural therapies can play in treating and preventing cystitis. Whilst antibiotics can be a necessary and important tool in fighting serious infection, when overused they can sometimes lead to a serious undermining effect in the body.

Cystitis falls into two categories – uncomplicated and complicated.

- *Uncomplicated UTI:* an uncomplicated UTI is relatively brief, usually lasting no longer than seven days. Symptoms include pain, frequency and urgency – even with an empty bladder – and pain and pressure in the pelvic area. Even if the infection is acute, a patient with an uncomplicated UTI won't usually have a fever and their underlying health will be generally good.

- *Complicated UTI*: a complicated UTI arises where a person has a separate condition or has undergone therapy which can cause, or lead to, infection in the bladder or urinary tract. Examples of these include diabetes, infections, immunosuppressive drugs, antibiotics, pregnancy and the use of a catheter or other urinary tract instrument.

Hormonal imbalances, such as a lack of oestrogen, can cause a thinning of the tissues in the vagina and urethra. This can make the occurrence of UTIs from opportunistic bacteria such as *E. coli* more likely to take hold.

Events that create a hormone imbalance by reducing the levels of oestrogen are many and varied. They include sexual intercourse, pregnancy, the menopause, spermicides, diaphragms, hormonal contraceptives and the pill.

Diagnosing UTIs

In most cases, GPs can diagnose UTIs simply from a patient's symptoms and a physical examination. Urine tests can also determine the presence of an infection while also ruling out sexually transmitted diseases and infections in the vagina. The urine test provided by the NHS is designed to give quick results and detect the presence of the most common bacteria associated with UTIs. It won't detect PBS, however, so a negative result from a urine analysis is likely to leave you none the wiser. For this reason, researchers specialising in UTIs have developed the urine broth culture.

WARNING

In some cases, UTIs can lead to a kidney infection. Initial symptoms of this are a fever and pain in the lower back. Infections in the kidney are serious and require early medical intervention. Do not attempt to treat a kidney infection at home, but always under the supervision of a practitioner.

The natural approach to UTIs

If you want to stay away from antibiotics (and who wouldn't?) there are several simple measures that you can take to help prevent UTIs and, in the unfortunate event that you develop one, overcome it. Remember, people with PBS can – and frequently do – develop UTIs so the following are useful guidelines for good bladder maintenance for all.

Prevention

- Drink enough fluid; for most people this should be about 2½ litres a day. The idea that drinking leads to more painful urination during the life of a UTI is not true. It is, in fact, the undiluted, infected urine that causes the most discomfort in the bladder and pain when urinating.

- Wear loose-fitting underwear made from natural materials: cotton, silk and hemp. Avoid synthetic fabrics as they make you sweat. Heat and moisture increase the growth of bacteria and fungus.

- Avoid chemical exposure from chemical soaps, shampoos and conditioners. Use unperfumed soaps. Never use bubble bath (a common cause of UTIs) as it can irritate the urethra and disrupts the healthy pH.

- Many people can feel when they are on the brink of getting an infection. This is the ideal time to take D-mannose (see page 28) and in many cases it is able to prevent the infection from developing.

- Probiotics help to maintain optimum gut flora and boost the body's immune system. Having a healthy balance of bacteria can be very important in preventing a UTI.

- Cut down on alcohol, citrus fruits, tea, coffee, tomatoes, vinegar, sugar and coffee. These are known bladder irritants and increase the risk of your developing a UTI.

- Consider your contraception – if you're worried about the effects of the pill, spermicides or hormonal contraceptives on your immunity to cystitis, change to a non-chemical method.

- Urinate after intercourse – this will help to clear the vaginal passage and genital area of any substance that may reinfect the area or compromise the vaginal flora. This is also the case for guys.

- Go when you need to – don't ignore the call of nature. Resisting the urge to urinate simply holds fluid in your bladder for longer than is necessary, increasing the likelihood of infection. When you feel the urge, urinate as soon as possible.

- Pay meticulous attention to hygiene. After a bowel movement, women should wash from front to back to avoid bacteria entering into the urethra.

- Cranberry can be a mixed blessing. Cranberry juice can help prevent infections,[6] as it is believed that it stops bacteria from adhering to the urinary tract. However, cranberries aren't necessarily helpful once you have an infection. Many people with PBS actually find cranberries aggravating to their bladder so they are contraindicated and not advisable.

Treatment

There are a number of natural botanical herbs that I have used to successfully treat UTIs. As well as being non-invasive, there are treatments that work quickly and can clear the infection. However, before taking any herbal remedies you should consult a suitably qualified practitioner.

The main herbs are listed in Table 5.2 on pages 84–91, though I also usually recommend a supplement known as D-mannose. This is a naturally occurring sugar, which finds its way to the urinary tract where it breaks the bond between *E. coli* and the bladder wall, enabling the body to flush out the *E. coli* through urination. D-mannose can be an excellent natural alternative to antibiotics.

WARNING

Although the herbal approach when correctly prescribed can be safe and entirely natural, always consult a trained herbalist or medical practitioner before starting any regime. Every person's circumstances are different and we all respond differently to different therapies. Your herbalist will be able to recommend the right blend and dosage of herbs specifically for you and adjust the regime as and when appropriate.

If you are sexually active and experiencing UTIs on a regular basis, it might be worth considering that you may be picking up bacterial infections from your partner. It might be worth them being tested for possible infections or at least being incredibly thorough with personal hygiene.

Val, age 42

Val kept getting cystitis. While it would clear up with antibiotics, it was never long before the condition returned. Although her GP was happy to continue prescribing the medication, Val's problem was a simple one: poor hydration. Her work, in a busy supermarket, prohibited Val from making frequent toilet breaks, so she kept her water intake to a minimum. As a result, Val wasn't sufficiently diluting her urine, so her bladder and urinary tract would become reinfected regularly.

Now, Val carries a water bottle which she sips from regularly and avoids leaving it too long before urinating when the need arises. She no longer gets cystitis. Sometimes the simple solutions are the most effective.

PBS and other conditions

Before we move on to the more positive aspects of treating PBS and developing strategies to enjoy a full and active life, I'd like to touch on another important aspect of the disease – its association with other conditions. PBS is frequently accompanied by one or more of a wide variety of overlapping conditions. These can include:

- autoimmune problems such as systemic lupus erythematosus (SLE), where the immune system mistakenly attacks its own healthy body tissue

- pelvic problems, including pelvic floor dysfunction

- vulvodynia – chronic pain in the vulva

- fibromyalgia – a painful musculoskeletal disorder

- chronic fatigue syndrome

- food allergies, including coeliac disease

- panic attacks.

It is also believed by many PBS researchers that people with irritable bowel syndrome (IBS), sensitive skin, endometriosis and a history of migraines are at increased risk of developing PBS.

CHAPTER 3

Conventional Painful Bladder Syndrome Treatment Methods

In this chapter, we'll look at some of the conventional drugs and treatments available to you if you have PBS. We'll also look at the role that diet can play in managing the condition. In both cases, however, there is no particular formula that suits everyone. Responses to specific drugs, therapies and dietary adjustments vary from person to person – even to the extent that what works for one individual can make symptoms worse for another!

Bear in mind also that the treatments and therapies described in this chapter are designed to alleviate your symptoms and help protect the damage that PBS/interstitial cystitis (IC) does to the bladder wall. Conventional medicine has not decided on an agreed or standardised treatment and these conditions are currently classified as incurable.

A range of drugs is available for PBS patients, aimed at relieving the symptoms of pain, frequency and inflammation and repairing the bladder wall.

Pain relief

Analgesics, both oral and in cream form for applying to the urethra or vulva area, are often used to alleviate pain, as are anti-inflammatories.

For chronic ongoing pain, you may be prescribed anticonvulsants or tricyclics/antidepressants. Amitriptyline, for example, prevents pain from travelling between the spinal cord and the brain. Some people report a sedative side-effect from amitriptyline, which aids sleep and relieves nocturia.

Frequency reduction

As well as amitriptyline, a group of medicines known as anticholinergics and antimuscarinics are available, which help to control bladder spasm and urge incontinence (the sudden need to urinate, often accompanied by leaking). Anticholinergics and antimuscarinics can increase bladder capacity, which in turn increases the intervals between toilet visits.

Inflammation relief

With PBS, inflammation of the bladder wall is often caused by histamines, the chemicals produced in allergic reactions. Some people obtain relief by taking antihistamines such as hydroxyzine (Atarax®), which can help with nocturia for a short time, and cimetidine (Tagamet®) which can alleviate PBS symptoms.[7] However, neither are without the risk of side-effects. Hydoxyzine can, amongst other reactions, cause impaired thinking and drowsiness. Some PBS patients experience gastrointestinal disturbance with cimetidine, such as nausea and diarrhoea.

A bladder installation can also have a direct effect on the bladder wall and potentially have an anti-inflammatory effect. An instillation involves the use of a specific drug, called an intravesical medication. A common one being

DMSO (dimethyl sulfoxide). The procedure involves instilling a solution directly into the bladder using a catheter for 15 minutes before voiding out. People can experience discomfort during the procedure and may also develop a garlicky taste for a few days. Some patients have also reported a burning sensation in the urethra when urinating, but these effects normally disappear within a day or two. If successful, treatment can be given every 14 days over a six- to eight-week period.

DMSO has been shown to have a detrimental effect on bladder muscles when used at high concentrations, and because of this the treatment is not as widely offered as it was.[8] Some patients, instead of feeling relief from the treatment, feel that it exacerbates their symptoms.

Bladder wall

As the breakdown of the glycosaminoglycan (GAG) layer, the protective lining of the bladder, seems to be at the root of PBS, protecting and repairing the bladder wall will be a large part of your treatment plan. There are currently a range of intravesical treatments, as well as the oral drug Elmiron®, which have been developed specifically for this purpose. I've listed some of these below, but if you want to try the conventional medical route then your urologist will be able to discuss which may be the most suitable for your specific symptoms.

Elmiron®

Also known also as pentosan polysulphate sodium, the oral medication Elmiron® is an anticoagulant which works by releasing itself from the urine onto the bladder wall, where it has a protective effect on the GAG layer. Some people need to allow anywhere between three weeks and six months before experiencing the effects of Elmiron®. Although available in the USA it is not a standard treatment option in the UK and is only prescribed on the NHS on a 'named patient' basis. Common side-effects include 'hair loss, diarrhoea, nausea, blood in the stool, headache, rash, upset stomach, abnormal liver function tests, dizziness and bruising'.[9]

Intravesical medications

These medications are placed directly into the bladder via a catheter and provide a protective coating to the bladder wall. Decisions regarding the suitability of these procedures must be taken by your urologist and most instillations should be performed by a qualified medical professional at a suitable outpatient clinic. No major side-effects are known to be associated with the instills described here, though the insertion of the catheter into the bladder may cause some localised irritation and there is an increased risk of infections.

IALURIL®

iAluRil® combines hyaluronic acid (1.6% w/v) and chondroitin sulphate (2.0% w/v), both of which occur naturally in a healthy GAG layer and elsewhere in the body including the heart valves, eye fluid, skin and joints. Once instilled into the bladder, these chemicals have a replenishing effect on the GAG layer, helping the bladder wall to recover and reform its protective lining. Treatments are often carried out weekly in month 1, fortnightly in month 2, and once monthly thereafter. Although usually administered by a nurse, you can be shown how to carry out the procedure yourself at home – a process known as self-catheterisation. With iAluRil® you can also repeat the initial course if you have a flare-up.

CYSTISTAT®

Cystistat contains sodium hyaluronate, a naturally occurring chemical in the GAG layer. When inserted into the bladder,

Cystistat® provides a temporary replacement GAG layer to the wall, relieving the symptoms of PBS. Treatments are often given weekly for the first four weeks, then monthly until symptoms disappear. All patients vary in their response time, but a good response can mean requiring repeat treatments at intervals of between six and twelve weeks. Up to six instillations may be needed before you notice any improvement. Usually a repeat of the treatment is offered if symptoms return.

GEPAN® INSTILL

The active ingredient in Gepan® instill is chondroitin sulphate (0.2%). Depending on your specific symptoms and your response to Gepan® instill, your urologist will recommend weekly instillations for four to six weeks, possibly followed by monthly procedures. Gepan® instill should be retained in the bladder for a minimum of 30 minutes, preferably as long as possible, while it replaces the GAG layer.

URACYST®

Uracyst® coats the damaged bladder wall with sterile sodium chondroitin sulphate solution (2.0%). This makes the lining waterproof again and helps to alleviate the pain, frequency and urgency of PBS. The instillation involves placing 20ml of the solution into the bladder and holding it in for a minimum of 30 minutes to achieve the best results. This takes place weekly for the first four to six weeks, then monthly until the symptoms desist. As with iAluRil®, it is possible to learn how to self-catheterise with Uracyst®.

HYACYST®

Hyacyst® coats the bladder wall with sodium hyaluronate, temporarily reducing inflammation and relieving pain, frequency and urgency. It is administered once weekly for the first four weeks, then once monthly until your symptoms are under control. Once instilled it should be held in for a minimum of half an hour – and preferably longer. Hyacyst® is available in two strengths, 40mg and 120mg, which means that your urologist can, if necessary, adjust your dosage without disrupting your treatment plan.

As you can see, there are a number of medical routes that can be taken in order to control the symptoms of PBS. However, many people choose to approach complimentary/alternative medical approaches not because of some philosophical bias towards natural medicine, but simply because the orthodox route hasn't worked for them.

CHAPTER 4

Holistic Medical Perspectives on the Causes of PBS

There is no definitive list of causes for PBS. However, as the disease is characterised by damage to the bladder lining, it is logical to believe that significant events in that area of the body can act as triggers and lead to its onset. Examples could be surgery or trauma in the spinal cord or pelvic area, bladder overdistention (such as when waiting too long to use a toilet) or problems with the pelvic floor muscles. Many experts also believe that autoimmune disorders, bacterial infections and hypersensitivity in the pelvic nerves are linked to PBS. Although there is ambiguity regarding the cause, I have, through clinical observation, established a link between gut health and PBS.

Inside inflammation

It is thought by a number of researchers that inflammation is at the root of many chronic diseases.[10] As well as being the major factor in PBS, it is thought by some to be the underlying cause of Alzheimer's, Parkinson's disease, arthritis, diabetes, heart disease, irritable bowel syndrome (IBS) and many other diseases. The suffix 'itis' means inflammation and cystitis is just one of a long list of diseases ending in these four letters. Researchers recently discovered a link between inflammation and cancer, while anyone with an allergy will have experienced inflammation in at least one part of the body as a result of exposure to a substance their body cannot tolerate. And, though the behaviours, symptoms and even names of these conditions vary greatly, the inflammatory process is, by comparison, constant. So much so in fact that the study of systemic, chronic inflammation has become as important – if not more so – as the research into the many diseases it gives rise to.

Inflammation is the body's initial response to injury, irritation or infection. When any of these events occur, blood flow to the affected area increases, carrying with it immune cells known as neutrophils, macrophages and phagocytes. The blood vessels become permeable, allowing the immune cells to pass through, surround the damaged tissue and deal with the unwelcome and harmful bacteria. They do this either by eating the invading toxins or by secreting hydrogen peroxide and other chemicals which kill them off, allowing them to be broken down and subsequently excreted. This increased blood flow and immune cell activity cause the area to heat up and become red. This is what we experience as inflammation, and it is a perfectly natural and healthy first response to external attacks on the body.

However, when inflammation becomes chronic – that is, when it stays around for a prolonged period of time – it becomes a disorder in itself. This is because after a while it moves on from attacking the invading toxins and bacteria to attacking the body's own healthy cells. This is known as an autoimmune response and it's what many researchers believe to be at the root of many degenerative and chronic diseases.

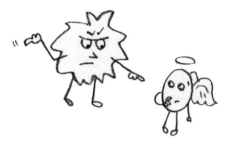

The gut connection

Many people who suffer with PBS also have digestive symptoms such as IBS, a condition characterised by symptoms of:

- abdominal pain and discomfort

- bloating

- wind

- irregular bowel movements, such as alternating between constipation and diarrhoea.

Research has shown that the majority of people with IBS and PBS have the presence of small intestine bacterial overgrowth.[11] This, as I will show, has significant implications for PBS sufferers with the gut being a fundamental piece of the puzzle.

With damage and inflammation to the bladder wall a defining feature of PBS, it follows that the more impurities there are in the urine, the more intensely its symptoms will be experienced. PBS is almost always accompanied by other conditions and, in every case I have treated, patients have also had leaky gut (also known as gut permeability syndrome). As its name suggests, leaky gut allows toxins and other undesirable substances to break through the lining of the gut wall with a wide range of consequences. One such consequence is that toxins generated from disturbed gut function may be processed by the liver and kidneys and end up in the bladder to be excreted.

Leaky gut or gut permeability syndrome is usually the result of an imbalance – or dysbiosis – of the gut flora, the composition of bacteria in the digestive system. Dysbiosis creates an environment in which 'bad' bacteria can multiply and overgrowths of yeasts such as *Candida albicans* can reach unmanageable levels. As it has major implications for people with PBS, it's worth taking a closer look at the causes and effects of leaky gut.

Seventy to 80 per cent of the body's immune cells are in our gut.[12] It is where the synthesis of vitamin B2 (riboflavin), vitamin B9 (folic acid), vitamin B12 (cobalamin), vitamin H (biotin) and vitamin K (phytomenadione) take place. Of all the organs in our body – including our skin – the gut has the largest surface area. And the job of this huge surface area is to provide a barrier to all manner of toxins, bacteria, heavy metals, petrochemicals and other undesirables. Helping to perform this function are a thick mucous membrane coating and some 100 trillion[13] bacteria of many different types. These bacteria combine with the tissue on tiny hairlike structures (microvilli) on the gut wall to synthesise immune system cells called lymphocytes.

Lymphocytes in turn produce antibodies known as immunoglobins, the most important of which is IgA (secretory immunoglobin A). Where the gut flora is healthy, IgA destroys unwanted viruses, bacteria, fungi, parasites and other impurities acquired through food and drink, vaccinations or the environment before they can do any damage to the digestive system. When dysbiosis occurs, however, the number of lymphocytes falls dramatically, reducing our capacity to produce IgA and weakening our natural immunity. To compound the problem, IgA antibodies are short-lived, so we need a healthy digestive system to slow their natural degradation down. Research is now indicating that gut flora regulate not only immune functions in the gut but also the entire immune system in the body.[14] Given that a healthy gut wall will provide around 85 per cent of our immunity, it's perhaps not surprising that it requires constant nourishment in the form of vitamins, minerals, amino acids and fats.

THE IMMUNE SYSTEM, GUT AND CAESAREAN SECTION

We are all born microbiologically sterile, that is, with no bacteria in our gut. During the first three days of our life, bacteria we ingest through a vaginal birth combine with the ingredients in the breast milk to colonise our gut flora. By the time we are two years old, our gut flora is fully developed.

Children born by caesarean section do not inherit this microbial environment.[15] They, along with non-breastfed babies, are more likely to develop allergies[16] and asthma[17] both in childhood and later life.

Probiotics developed for babies and adults can be very helpful in providing the necessary bacteria and building immunity in people born by caesarean section. The regular intake of probiotics can be enormously important for adults who were born by caesarean section and/or not breastfed.

Insufficient levels of good bacteria in the gut affect the immune system. One way that this happens is through a reduction in the effectiveness and numbers of neutrophils[18] and macrophages, whose role is to form around inflamed tissue and swallow and destroy viruses, toxins and harmful bacteria. Gut bacteria, such as lactobacillus, excrete a multitude of important substances, such as its own version of an antibiotic[19] (acidophilin) and beneficial acids, which make the intestine unsuitable for the growth of yeasts and fungus.[20] Another function of healthy gut flora is the production of active regulators of our immune response. By this I mean our natural ability to withstand exposure to viruses through vaccinations or the external environment and deal with them as a matter of routine. An abnormal gut flora, however, allows these viruses to survive undamaged within our bodies.

Known causes of leaky gut are extended exposure to antibiotics, painkillers, steroids, contraceptive pills, highly processed foods, over- or under-eating and disease or infection in the digestive system. Stress, in the short term, can do minor yet repairable damage to the gut, though over the long term its effect can be difficult to reverse. Other factors that can affect good bacteria are alcoholism, physical exertion, pollution, toxic metals, radiation, old age and extreme climates.

People unknowingly intolerant to certain foods – and in particular gluten, soy and dairy products – are also at risk of increased gut permeability. This is because these foods can, for some, cause inflammation of the gut wall and create openings for them to pass through undigested along with other harmful chemicals and microorganisms, triggering a response from the immune system. These sensitivities are what we know as food allergies.

Leaky gut also contributes to abnormal immune reactions. This is because abnormality in the flora causes the excessive production of our natural defence against allergies in the form of an antibody called immunoglobin E (IgE). IgE creates a histamine-type response which can prevent low-grade allergies from being detected. As well as the incorrect molecules from food passing through the intestinal wall and triggering immune reactions, malabsorption also occurs. Mineral and vitamin deficiencies, particularly zinc, magnesium, B6 and B12, can simultaneously develop.

HISTAMINE

Histamine is a chemical that we naturally produce and store in the body in small quantities. When we have an allergic reaction, for example to an insect bite, we produce histamine in increased quantity and send it to the affected area. Histamine triggers inflammation and facilitates an immune response to address any foreign invaders and infection. This creates the familiar allergy symptoms of rashes, itchiness, and so on. However, for some people the body produces excess of histamine unnecessarily, which results in allergies, such as to pollen or animal hair. A leaky gut, where bad bacteria are allowed to run riot, can amongst other factors lead to higher levels of histamine, a condition known as 'histadelia', a term coined by the psychiatrist Dr Carl Pfeiffer. Symptoms of histadelia include allergies, low blood pressure, excessive body fluids and hormonal changes. Patients can also experience emotional instability, addictions and abnormal sleep patterns. Conventional treatment for high histamine, such as prescribing antihistamines, tends to focus on the symptoms. However, a holistic approach would entail restoring healthy biochemistry by addressing nutrient deficiencies and measures to repair the gut lining.

To summarise then, leaky gut can result in nutrient deficiencies as well as preventing the body from fully separating harmful substances from nutrients at the point of digestion. Instead of being processed for excretion (see below), toxins, incompletely digested food and bacteria find their way into the bloodstream (translocation) causing immune and inflammatory responses in the body.[21, 22]

DIGESTION – WHAT SHOULD HAPPEN

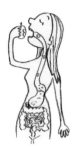

Consuming and processing food is a complex process and the subject of extensive research and medical study. However, to give you a bite-sized summary, the key stages are as follows:

1. Eating: as we chew our food, an enzyme in the saliva called amylase helps to break it down, making it possible to swallow.

2. Creating chyme: when the food reaches the stomach, hydrochloric acid and pepsin break down the proteins to produce chyme.

3. Digesting and separating: amalyse, protease and lipase are released by the pancreas to further digest protein and carbohydrates, while the gall bladder and liver excrete bile for the digestion of fats. All this takes place in the small intestine before nutrients and harmful substances part company – the former being absorbed through the microvilli on the gut wall, the latter being moved to the large intestine.*

4. Excreting: water gets absorbed from the chyme. The resulting solid substance, faeces, is excreted during a bowel movement.

> * This is where things go wrong with a leaky gut. Instead of being filtered out, many harmful substances also pass through the gut wall along with the nutrients, thus reducing their beneficial effects and putting the liver, kidneys, bladder and other organs under pressure.

Yeast overgrowth

Of all the microbes that can overgrow as a result of gut dysbiosis, the most commonly detected is a yeast known as Candida. There are several types of Candida, the most common being Candida albicans.

Candida exists in low levels in the human body, but its growth is kept in check by the beneficial bacteria in a healthy gut. As we have seen, abnormal gut flora leads to an absence of these friendly bacteria, opening the door to the overgrowth of Candida.

Candida belongs to a category known as opportunistic flora, so called because it takes advantage of factors that cause the gut to become compromised. Antibiotics, for example, are known killers of good bacteria, but other medication can disrupt the delicate balance of bacteria by other means; for example, proton pump inhibitors – medications designed to reduce the amount of acid produced in the stomach, making the pH more alkaline. This also means that potentially harmful bacteria and fungi in food don't get killed off in the stomach, making infection more likely in the small intestine.[23] Other factors leading to yeast overgrowth include steroids, the chlorine in our tap water and heavy metals such as mercury. How does mercury get into the digestive system? If you have mercury fillings in your teeth, there's a good chance that offgassing (the release and subsequent inhalation of vapour from those fillings) will allow traces of the metal to enter your gut and compromise the balance of bacteria.

Higher than manageable levels of Candida lead to a number of unpleasant conditions. These include thrush and yeast-based cystitis. Further complications arise, as it is thought that Candida is able to produce the toxins acetaldehyde and ethanol through fermenting sugars in the gut.[24] Again, neither of these would cause undue distress in a healthy gut, but where flora is compromised, the body is ill-equipped to control the behaviours of these contaminants. Acetaldehyde is thought to affect red blood cells and interfere with neurotransmitters, the chemicals that transmit signals through the body. Tell-tale signs of dangerous levels of acetaldehyde are fatigue, drowsiness and the feeling of having been poisoned. Another effect is the hindering of liver detoxification pathways. This can lead to 'multiple chemical sensitivity', in which inflammation and other symptoms appear in response to a normally harmless exposure to chemicals, for example wet paint. Ethanol meanwhile is an alcohol – and I'm sure most readers will be aware of what having too much of that in the system feels like. Unfortunately, these same effects can be felt when ethanol proliferates in the system – and all that without even having a drink! More seriously, ethanol can also induce neurological and psychiatric problems.

Yeast overgrowth usually accompanies leaky gut and is associated with abdominal conditions such as nausea and, in particular, IBS, a disorder that most people with PBS are also likely to have. As well as being a consequence of leaky gut, Candida exacerbates the condition: yeast compromises the gut lining, increasing its permeability. This leads to the by-products of Candida and the digestive process infiltrating the gut epithelium and entering the bloodstream, increasing the load on the liver's detoxification ability.

Dysbiosis and yeast overgrowth are more likely if you have an insufficiency of stomach acid, which is critical to the healthy functioning of the digestive system.

Detecting an overgrowth of Candida in the gut is possible by way of an extensive stool analysis. The UK's National Health Service (NHS) does not offer this service as a matter of routine but, if you are concerned that you may have yeast overgrowth, you can arrange a test through a private practitioner who will organise it with a laboratory.

Leanne, age 35

Leanne had had problems with bloating and wind since her late teens, experiencing the extremes of constipation and loose stools and everything in between. Although things would often get worse around her periods, the bloating was ever-present.

Ever since she can remember, Leanne had a tendency to cystitis, and frequently felt on the verge of the next infection. Despite taking antibiotics, her symptoms invariably worsened and would be followed by long-lasting episodes of thrush.

Then Leanne learned about Candida overgrowth and the links between her medical history – which included a lot of antibiotics as a child and teenager –and her current condition became clear.

She eliminated the usual aggravants, such as wheat, dairy, sugar and yeast, from her diet and added grapefruit seed extract capsules and probiotics. For about two weeks following the change, she felt rotten due to the yeast dying off and releasing its poisons into the body. However, by the third week, she had the bloating fully under control and no longer felt heavy after eating.

The sense of impending cystitis disappeared after two months. Leanne's moods became much more stable and even her period pains became more bearable.

Stomach acid

Hydrochloric acid (HCl) in the stomach plays a critical role in food digestion and it is vital that we produce it in the correct quantities. Its role is to break down proteins into amino acids ready for digestion by the enzyme, pepsin, and to kill bad bacteria, viruses, yeast and fungi. The healthy pH level of HCl in the stomach needs to be between 1.8 and 2.6. This is highly acidic – enough to attack the stomach wall itself if it wasn't for its mucous coating and certainly enough to burn naked skin. However, this high acidity also protects us from food poisoning and infections such as *E. coli*, which cannot survive below pH 3.5.

It follows then that when HCl levels are low (hypochlorida) or non-existent (achlorida), the absorption of proteins and our defence against infections are severely compromised, leading to a whole range of effects on our health and wellbeing.

HCl is produced by cells in the stomach lining called parietal cells. The efficiency of parietal cells naturally drops as we age, starting with a gradual reduction of secretion around the age of 50, followed by a more marked decline throughout our 60s and 70s. Our capability to produce sufficient levels of HCl can also be affected by alcohol, stress, rushed eating and drinking, low levels of zinc, antibiotics, offgassing from mercury amalgam fillings and Candida overgrowth. Some people may have a genetic predisposition to low HCl production.

Prescribed medications for the relief of indigestion and gastric reflux – proton pump inhibitors – also lower the production of HCl and consequently the pH level of the stomach acid.

Certain combinations of herbs as well as adequate levels of zinc, combined with a regular eating routine, all help to restore healthy levels of acid in the stomach. In

Part II I'll be explaining how to incorporate these into a holistic PBS management programme. However, you might spot the paradox. Acidic foods can aggravate the condition of someone with PBS, yet we are looking, if insufficient, to increase stomach acidity. When the stomach acid pH is insufficient, inadequate quantities and concentration of acidity-neutralising digestive fluids are produced. This ultimately results in acid food not being sufficiently neutralised, therefore too much acid getting into the gut and reaching the bladder.

THE STOMACH ACID TEST

First thing in the morning, on an empty stomach before eating or drinking anything, stir a quarter of a teaspoon of bicarbonate of soda into 250ml of water. Drink the mixture, then, using a stopwatch, time how long it takes to start belching.

1 to 2 minutes indicates a normal HCl level

2 to 3 minutes suggests you have a normal to slightly low HCl level

3 to 5 minutes signals hypochlorida – a low HCl level

over 5 minutes is a sign that you have achlorida, no HCl at all.

The belching is caused by carbon dioxide gas, the result of a chemical reaction between the HCl and the bicarbonate of soda.[25]

As well as depriving the body of vital proteins and brain chemicals and exposing us to infections and food poisoning, hypochlorida and achlorida usually lead to vitamin, mineral and amino acid deficiencies.

Furthermore, without the required acidity level in the stomach, we lose some of our defence against parasites, yeasts, fungi and bacteria. Should we fall prey to any of these invaders, symptoms of poor digestion, including diarrhoea, are likely to follow.

Having the correct level of HCl is also essential for the production of intrinsic factor – a substance which enables us to absorb B12. As I will cover later on, B12 is incredibly important for our physical and mental health. When I test PBS patients for B12, they tend to have a deficiency. The relevance is apparent as B12 deficiency can lead to neurological conditions, bladder incontinence, recurrent cystitis, neurogenic bladder, as well as delayed wound healing, such as ongoing ulceration.[26]

And, as we have seen, poorly digested foods affect the flora in the gut, starting a chain of events that invariably lead to leaky gut.

So what does leaky gut mean for the bladder?

As I have discussed, when the gut flora is abnormal, the epithelial lining of the intestinal wall becomes compromised. The gut wall becomes increasingly permeable, allowing toxins and insufficiently digested food to pass through it. In a compromised gut, certain substances such as acetaldehyde can become potent immune aggravators. And in this scenario gliadin, a protein found in gluten-containing grains, is even implicated in creating an autoimmune response in the body, the toxic effects of which enter the bloodstream and are carried into the liver, which is now presented with an unmanageable burden.

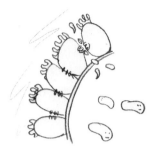

The problem is two-fold in that (a) both the gut and liver are under enormous extra pressure and (b) the digestive system is struggling to break down foods and provide the nourishment these organs need to do their jobs. The result is that neurotoxic debris that the liver is unable to deal with passes through to the kidneys and into the bladder. This I believe is how many cases of PBS begin. Once the bladder lining is damaged, particles in the urine begin to find their way in and cause further complications, including chronic nerve pain. Under normal circumstances, the bladder lining usually repairs itself and the symptoms disappear. For people with PBS/interstitial cystitis (IC), however, this is often not the case. The current thinking on the reasons for this is that PBS patients produce a protein called APF (antiproliferative factor), which prevents the growth of healthy replacement bladder cells.[27]

The liver

So far, we've seen how abnormal flora, yeast overgrowths and insufficient levels of hydrochloric acid in the stomach can compromise the gut wall. When the gut's defences are breached, the liver becomes vulnerable. Among the liver's known 500 functions is detoxification, a major factor in bladder health and, therefore, highly relevant to PBS.

Situated on the right of the body beneath the rib cage, the liver is the heaviest single organ we have. It filters almost all of our blood every three to four minutes, a process which helps to absorb the healthy parts of what we eat and drink and detoxify the rest. This involves cleaning the blood and removing bacteria, man-made chemicals, drugs and toxins such as caffeine and alcohol.

As part of its Herculean work rate, the liver also:

- maintains a healthy hormonal balance by producing and breaking down oestrogen and testosterone

- produces co-factors which allow oestrogen and other hormones to work properly

- metabolises proteins and carbohydrates to produce energy

- stores and assimilates vitamins, minerals and sugars

- produces bile, which helps to break down fats

- produces immune-enhancing substances

- produces up to one litre of digestive fluids a day

- breaks down adrenalin and cortisol, chemicals we produce when we experience stress, anxiety and emotional pressure.

The liver converts chemicals from a fat-soluble to water-soluble form. This makes it possible for us to pass them through urine, sweat or faeces.

When the liver is healthy, we enjoy good digestion, rarely get bloated and can take moderate levels of stress in our stride. Conversely, a diseased liver will make itself known via symptoms such as inflammation, jaundice, gall bladder pain and cirrhosis. These symptoms are acutely felt and easy to identity. The problem for many people, including those with PBS, is that there is a middle ground between a healthy and diseased liver which conventional medicine rarely picks up on. Indications that the liver is operating in this grey area are headaches, acid reflux from fatty foods, nausea, skin problems and irritability. In most cases, we're prescribed an over-the-counter product to suppress the symptoms and encouraged to think little more of it.

These symptoms, however, are often the liver's way of telling us that things are not 100 per cent right. In this scenario, treating the symptoms only – such as taking a paracetamol every time we have a headache – makes things worse. Also complicating the diagnosis of liver disorders is the fact that, in many cases, the underlying problem can reach an advanced stage before symptoms are severe. An example of this is hepatitis C, with which patients may feel tired but could go many years before experiencing any direct liver symptoms.

Liver detoxification pathways

Where symptoms suggest that the liver is not functioning at optimum efficiency, appropriate liver support can help to get things back on track. How to prepare a liver flush at home is described in the Appendix. First, though, let's examine the liver detoxification process.

The liver has two main detoxification pathways, Phase I and Phase II:

- *Phase I*: Phase I is where fat-soluble toxins are transformed into a water-soluble form, enabling them to be neutralised and excreted harmlessly through the route of the kidneys. This complicated series of processes is carried out by P450 enzymes. Toxins that cannot be completely neutralised by this stage are partly processed; however, they are, until they reach Phase II, highly unstable and can be temporarily more toxic.

- *Phase II*: Phase II rids the liver of toxins produced in Phase I. In a process called conjugation, the toxins are combined with sulphur and acids before being excreted in bile.

Some toxins will be rendered harmless by a single phase alone; others have to undergo both Phase I and Phase II. For this reason, both phases must be effective for the liver to fully detoxify. And to achieve this, we rely on a complex series of enzyme processes. In Phase I, the most common enzyme is also the most powerful of them all. Known as Cytochrome P450, it remains unaffected by chemical drugs and pollutants.

Phase II uses a compound called glutathione, a powerful antioxidant created by the synthesis of three amino acids, cysteine, glutamine and glycine. Though present in every cell, glutathione, which is reliant on sulphur in our diet, is at its most concentrated in the liver. However, concentration levels here can drop if there are large quantities of toxins to metabolise. Viruses, bacterial infections, alcohol and recreational drugs also deplete the store of glutathione. Needless to say, detoxification suffers when levels are low.

Toxins that go through both phases are broken down in Phase I, ready for conjugation in Phase II. At this stage they are sometimes even more toxic than in their original form. Sulphur and glutathione are required in the right quantities at this stage. If there is a deficiency, detoxification is compromised and free radical levels can rise.

The interaction between liver and kidney/bladder

The filtration and detoxification pathways of the liver are of key importance to kidney and bladder health. Compromised liver pathways can mean that toxins which are not neutralised can still get to the kidneys. Although the kidneys are an incredibly efficient filtration system, they do not have the capability of neutralising toxins. The only option the kidneys then have is to quickly expel them via the bladder and urinary tract, although inevitably tissue damage and irritation can be the result, as someone with PBS is all too familiar with. Tissue that is irritated and inflamed is then much more vulnerable to infection.

Factors in liver health

Several factors influence the health of the liver, as described below.

FATS

While certain fats are an essential part of our diet, there are many others that can cause harm. The main culprits are fried and heated oils (the high cooking heat changes their structure), oils that have gone rancid, hydrogenated products (their chemical makeup is similar to plastic) and trans fats.

Harmful fats are thought to increase cholesterol levels. Although cholesterol is naturally produced in the liver to protect arteries, the common medical understanding is that quantities need to be kept in check. Cholesterol and its role in health, however, is actually much more complicated than we first thought. It was thought that too much cholesterol caused by eating too much fat can block the arteries, which can lead to heart disease. However, it isn't as simple as that. Cholesterol is essential for a healthy body as well as a healthy mind. Cholesterol is an important component for healthy cells, and particularly the cell membrane. It is an essential building block needed by the body to create hormones such as testosterone and adrenal hormones such as cortisol. Research has shown that cholesterol's presence in the body can even act like an antioxidant.[28] Cholesterol has even been shown to prevent infection through enhanced immune response and have a protective effect against the development of arteriosclerosis (hardening of the arteries).[29] A link has also been identified between lower total cholesterol levels and an increased risk of urinary tract infections in both men and women.[29]

In the 1950s, high cholesterol levels began to be observed in people with coronary heart disease.[30] With these findings it was then thought that reducing the cholesterol level would reduce the incidence of heart disease. However, a study reported in the *British Medical Journal* concluded that:

> Lowering serum cholesterol concentrations does not reduce mortality and is unlikely to prevent coronary heart disease.[31]

Confusing…yes? The more you delve into the subject of cholesterol the more complex and increasingly contradictory it seems.

Either way, we do know that cholesterol is present at higher concentrations when there is inflammation in the body. However, it could be that high cholesterol is a sign that the body is in a state of chronic inflammation, and is regulating the production of cholesterol in order to actually deal with the inflammation because of the enhanced immune function that this provides.

Chronic inflammation in our body can be caused by many factors, amongst which are the usual suspects: heavy metals, smoking, environmental toxins, toxic metabolites that have been inadequately processed because of compromised detoxification pathways and a diet high in sugar and refined carbohydrates.

The standard medical approach has been to lower cholesterol levels by any means necessary, whether through diet or through drugs. However, cholesterol is also needed by the brain to function properly and is fundamental to the structure of the nervous system and myelin sheath. Low blood cholesterol levels have been associated with low brain serotonin levels and risk of 'suicidal, violent, and impulsive behaviour'.[32]

One of conventional medicine's responses to high cholesterol levels is a drug type known as statins. Statins shut down some of the liver functions associated with cholesterol production. However, they can also reduce the production of CoQ10,[33] an important enzyme which is involved in energy production in the body.

Fat is important in our diet for the repair of our gut lining, and saturated fat, although portrayed as the 'bad guy', is fundamental to the repair process.

CHEMICALS AND DRUGS

Liver damage is a potential side-effect of most prescription drugs. The effects of recreational drugs and chemicals in the environment such as pesticides and formaldehyde are even worse, ranging from liver toxicity to the destruction of liver cells. Those with PBS often notice an exacerbation of symptoms when taking prescription drugs, and pain medication in the form of aspirin or paracetamol being a common aggravate. Steroidal medication and antihistamine medication also seem to cause side-effects for many. As you may already know too well, almost anything can aggravate a PBS bladder, and it is important to be vigilant, as sometimes there can be a delayed response, with a flare-up arising hours and even days after consuming a medication or a food.

Where the liver is under a heavy toxic burden, chemicals are put aside as part of a backlog to be dealt with at a later date. This allows them to attach themselves to fats and remain in the body, potentially for years. A programme of rapid weight loss will release these toxins causing headaches, insomnia and irritability, and if very toxic chemicals are released could be very dangerous, for example for people who have had significant toxic exposure such as chemotherapy or organophosphates. Any potential weight loss programme must be very gradual so that the body does not get overwhelmed and cause further problems.

ALCOHOL

When we consume alcohol, for the body to process it the liver enzymes first convert it into the even more toxic chemical, acetaldehyde. This is when we experience the symptoms of a hangover, such as a headache. Acetaldehyde goes through the liver detoxification pathways described above, where it is converted into acetic acid, which is easier to deal with. High alcohol consumption causes high levels of acetaldehyde, some of which then leaks into the bloodstream. From here it can affect the neurotransmitters in the brain. The inability of the body to convert this surplus acetaldehyde into acetic acid exposes us to the risk of alcohol poisoning. In some populations, including indigenous peoples and East Asians, up to 50 per cent of people are genetically unable to convert acetaldehyde into acetic acid, and therefore cannot metabolise alcohol. They experience toxic reactions causing nausea, headaches, dizziness and facial flushing. For PBS patients alcohol in all forms is a particularly aggressive irritant, and usually needs to be absolutely avoided whilst on a recovery programme.

Sluggish liver

A 'sluggish liver' or 'liver stagnation' is a term often used by holistic practitioners to describe a situation in which the detox pathways are not fully functioning. When the ordinary internal metabolic and external environmental toxins do not get adequately neutralised, all kinds of seemly unrelated conditions can arise – anything from headaches and inflammatory skin conditions such as psoriasis, acne and eczema to hormonal and digestive imbalances.

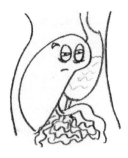

Other symptoms of a sluggish liver are:

* tiredness in the morning
* allergies
* bitter or bad taste in the mouth
* eye problems
* poor digestion of fatty foods
* irritability
* headaches and migraines
* mood swings
* hormonal imbalances
* sensitivity to environmental factors such as perfume, paints and odours.

A sluggish liver affects hormonal balances in both sexes. It can intensify the symptoms of premenstrual tension in women and compromise the metabolism of testosterone, causing excess supplies in men and women. This can lead to irritability, aggression and irregular sexual energy.

Healing the liver

Despite the perpetual onslaught the liver can face from the modern world and the western diet, its powers of recuperation are remarkable. It can withstand the removal of up to 75 per cent of its tissue during surgery and still restore itself to its original size.

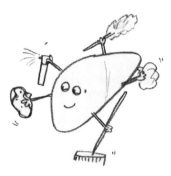

Given its vital role in so many processes – not least, preventing toxins from entering the urine and, by extension, the bladder – taking the time to cleanse the liver is well worthwhile as this helps to:

- maximise the efficiency of the detoxification pathways
- protect the liver from any additional damage
- ensure healthy bowel movements.

We'll look at some simple yet effective ways to cleanse the liver and maintain the health of this vital organ in Part II.

Stress and adrenal fatigue

Stress and emotional trauma are major obstructions to the body's healing processes. Although conventional medicine tends to categorise stress as a purely mental or psychological problem, it has definite physiological implications that affect our ability to manage illness.

Located on each kidney are the adrenal glands. As their name suggests, they produce adrenalin and noradrenalin, the hormones we feel coursing through our bodies in moments of panic and fear. The adrenal glands also produce cortisol, which in turn raises blood sugar. This helps us cope with emergencies and other mentally, emotionally and physically demanding situations. Another substance produced by the adrenal glands is dehydroepiandrosterone (DHEA). Relatively little is known about DHEA, though it is associated with bone and muscle health and general vitality, and is involved with controlling inflammation, immunity and sexual function. Research is also showing that declining levels of DHEA is related to mental decline as we get older.[34]

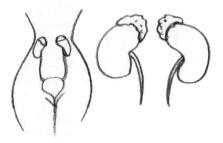

Together, these chemicals provide our flight, fight or freeze response – our often involuntary reactions to extreme threats to our safety. Thankfully, for most people, such events are relatively rare these days; however, these same bodily functions are activated by something far more prevalent in the modern world: stress.

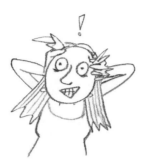

We all experience stress at some time in our lives – and indeed in small doses it can have a positive effect. At manageable levels, our body responds to stress by releasing increased levels of cortisol to get us through our immediate predicament, then returns to normal production levels. This response is made possible by the hypothalamic-pituitary-adrenal axis (HPA), a complex set of connections and neurotransmitters that allow instructions to pass from the pituitary gland in the head down to the adrenal glands.

Problems begin to arise – and multiply – when we are subject to stress on a prolonged basis, something that many people in all walks of life will recognise. Ongoing stress means the ongoing production of cortisol at unnaturally high levels. Eventually the body will regard this high level as the norm and produce excess cortisol as a matter of course. This is known as adrenal hyperactivity and can lead to a wide range of symptoms including weight gain, excess perspiration and problems with hair and skin. Too much cortisol can also reduce bone density.

While under this increased cortisol-producing workload, the adrenal glands' capacity to produce DHEA becomes compromised, resulting in general fatigue, loss of libido and a general lack of motivation.

If this isn't unsettling enough, a third problem awaits. Depending on each individual's circumstances, underlying health and the type and level of stress he or she is exposed to, the adrenal glands eventually tire under the strain of excess cortisol production. When this happens, cortisol levels nosedive, leaving an undersupply of cortisol and DHEA in the body. The patient now has adrenal hypoactivity, or adrenal fatigue, and is feeling the topsy-turvy effects of the transition from a cortisol oversupply to a cortisol deficiency – with no happy medium in between. DHEA levels also remain low. The symptoms already in play are likely now to be compounded by irregular sleep patterns, mild depression and a sense of being overwhelmed by what are, under normal circumstances, the routine rhythms of life. When this happens we are truly running on empty, and may feel tired and wired.

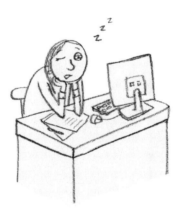

Irregular sleep patterns, in particular, cause problems for adrenal wellbeing. This is because healthy cortisol production is at its highest around one hour after we wake up and gradually drops throughout the day and evening. So, a person working regular office hours who wakes up at, say, 4.00am and is unable to get back to sleep will be feeling the effects of declining cortisol levels even before the working day gets started. Some people with adrenal fatigue report that they feel more awake in the evening than they do in the morning – a classic sign that their cortisol production has become irregular. Similarly, people with lifestyles or working patterns (such as shift working) that result in irregular sleeping times are also at risk of adrenal fatigue.

It is possible to test adrenal health by analysing saliva. I frequently carry out this test with new patients who complain of tiredness and low libido. Unsurprisingly, their cortisol and DHEA production are often flatlining – a sure sign of adrenal fatigue.

If left unattended, the longer-term risks of adrenal fatigue include longer recovery times from inflammation and illness and shorter life expectancy.

Annie, age 42

Annie is a marketing executive with a busy and often stressful job. Her life involves frequent meetings, working lunches and overseas travel. In the period leading up to her symptoms her eating and sleeping patterns were irregular. The only real constants in her daily life were coffee and cigarettes.

Annie's problems started suddenly, on a long haul flight to Hong Kong. Out of nowhere she felt a pain in her kidney area and developed a high fever. She was aware that she hadn't drunk much liquid on the flight, but this was a new sensation, quite unlike any previous bouts of cystitis in the past. By the time the flight landed Annie was feeling ill and couldn't urinate. Unable to even continue her journey, Annie checked into a hospital where she was told she had a serious kidney infection and a temperature of 39 degrees. By this time, even walking was difficult.

Annie spent the next five days in hospital and was put on intravenous antibiotics. Once she was up and walking again she went straight back into her hectic work schedule. Unsurprisingly, a month later she was unwell again: her kidney ached, she felt nauseous and was running a high temperature. Recognising the symptoms, Annie went back onto antibiotics.

The cycle continued over several months, with the pain always going to Annie's kidneys rather than the urinary tract or the bladder. After the fifth infection, she knew she had to break the cycle.

Annie consulted a naturopath, who carried out an adrenal saliva hormone test. This revealed low levels of cortisol, indicating that Annie had been running on empty for far too long. A radical change of lifestyle followed: Annie quit smoking, cut the alcohol and coffee from her diet and started going to bed before midnight. Her naturopath also recommended a blend of herbs as part of her new regime.

One of the herbs that really helped Annie was liquorice, which helps restore adrenal function. She also took probiotics to replace bacteria that had been stripped from her gut, leading to frequent episodes of thrush.

Despite a small blip over Christmas, when Annie overdid things and got a minor infection, she has been symptom-free for two years. And even though her adrenal score remains at the lower end of the scale she is well equipped to control her health.

Dealing with stress

Stress is not usually caused by any particular event; it is caused by the way we react to that event. In other words, it is our own individual response to the disparity between 'what we want to happen and what is actually happening'. What triggers stress varies from person to person; what may cause anxiety or irritability in one may be casually laughed off by another, and vice-versa.

Ancient medical systems such as Ayurveda from India or Chinese medicine have many strategies that help with preventing the damaging effects of stress and the recovery from adrenal fatigue. Key areas to consider are:

- Routine; this is incredibly important to restore the natural rhythm and cycles. It's about eating at the same time every day, getting up at the same time, going to bed on time, and living a lifestyle that is sustainable. This is one of the most important steps to restoring your capacity to heal.

- When we are fatigued, a certain amount of exercise can be helpful, but not to the extent where we are overexerting ourselves.

- Find a way to centre yourself as a way of dealing with stressful situations. This could be mindfulness meditation, tai chi, yoga, walking, dancing. Find something which doesn't aggravate your PBS and works for you.

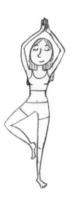

What is constant is that a great deal of stress stays with us, even after the stressful event is behind and our mood has changed. We store all sorts of stress, from emotional trauma and post-traumatic stress disorder (PTSD) to a whole range of unresolved trauma, possibly dating back many years, in the muscles in our body. One of the muscles most commonly affected by stored stress seems to be the psoas muscle.

THE PSOAS MUSCLE

The psoas is one of the largest and thickest muscles we have. Beginning at the 12th thoracic vertebra, it runs down the mid- and lower spine, connecting to all the vertebral bodies and discs, the lumbar vertebrae and the pelvis and attaching to the inside of the top of the leg. Its main job is to flex the spine and the hip and provide the fluid motion to our gait.

The psoas also supports our abdominal organs and acts as a hydraulic pump that works with the diaphragm to massage our internal organs.

When faced with a life or death situation the fight, flight or freeze response kicks in. Under extreme stress it is instinctive either to lie down in the embryo position – knees bent toward the chest, back bent forward – or crouch down in a similar pose to protect our facial features and reproductive organs. This posture involves the contraction of the psoas muscle. So ingrained is this response to panic that the psoas muscle will contract whenever we experience stress, anxiety or emotional trauma. So, a person experiencing stress over an extended period of time will have regular contractions of his or her psoas muscle. Over time, this will shorten the psoas and this can lead to lower back pain, poor posture and other related conditions.

The body's natural response to trauma is to shake. When we are children and have a traumatic experience, we shake for some time afterwards. This is the body's way of discharging all the excess energy caused by the fight, flight or freeze hormones and restoring normality. As we grow older, however, we become conditioned by a perceived social stigma attached to the outward display of fear and anxiety and develop strategies to suppress this shaking. And by doing so, we lock trauma and stress inside our body.

Most people have some degree of trauma, either emotional or physical, in their history and certainly most of the PBS patients I see carry this around with them in their body. (In the USA a recent study found that between 18 and 33% of people with PBS have been sexually abused at some point in their life.) Once we can release this trauma from the body, we can begin to benefit from increased flow of qi (energy) through the body. And because the psoas is located close to the bladder, releasing stress and trauma stored in this muscle, when done carefully, helps PBS patients enormously.

Sita, age 29

Despite frequent urination and chronic fatigue, Sita's case of PBS was diagnosed as relatively mild. However, her fatigue would kick in early in the afternoon and she would often be in bed by 4.00pm.

Improvements in her diet helped to moderate Sita's energy fluctuations, but not enough to improve her overall stamina.

To help increase her energy, Sita began working with a massage therapist/body worker. During her sessions it emerged that bereavements in her past had stored high levels of trauma in her body. Sita's father passed away when she was in her early teens and her sister died in a car crash when Sita was in her early twenties. In effect, the trauma had blocked the flow of qi through Sita'a body, preventing healing processes from having a meaningful effect.

Sita's body worker showed her a few exercises that she could do at home. These encouraged shaking to start releasing the trauma held in her body.

Once she had become adept at shaking exercises, Sita felt something suddenly change about 20 minutes into one of her sessions. She reported a warm sensation and a feeling of connection with her body that she had never experienced before. Through regular shaking exercises, Sita was able to release the shock held in her body. In turn, she rediscovered her energy levels and was soon able to stay up throughout the evenings without the debilitating fatigue. The frequent urination calmed down, and although it sometimes recurs at times of acute stress, Sita believes she has conquered the worst symptoms of PBS.

As I will discuss later, shaking is a traditional method of releasing trauma as well as stuck mental and emotional patterns. Many indigenous cultures use shaking as a way of clearing stagnation and blockages. In qigong, an ancient Chinese whole body exercise to improve health, shaking is often done to stimulate the healing potential of the body. Many ancient shamanic practices were developed over the millennia as a way of dealing with and releasing trauma and of assisting the healing process when it was blocked. Talking therapies can be incredibly helpful as a way of understanding ourselves and others, whereas body-orientated approaches are a very direct way to encourage healing and resolution.

To introduce this concept I will explain some very simple exercises that are recommended by trauma therapists as a way of physically releasing body distress. These are designed to bring about shaking, the body's natural expulsion mechanism that, for social reasons, we have learned to resist. In Part II, I will explore in detail some very simple exercises that are recommended by trauma therapists as a way of physically releasing body distress. These are designed to bring about shaking, the body's natural expulsion mechanism which, for social reasons, we have learned to resist.

Teething problems

Another place where problems can start – and lead to the worsening of PBS symptoms – is the mouth. There are several dental and oral health conditions that have implications for the gut and, by extension, the liver and the bladder. By far the most significant of these is the presence of mercury.

Mercury – the menace in the mouth

Mercury is a heavy metal. Unlike other metals such as zinc, copper and iron which, in small quantities, are essential to our health, mercury has no place in the human body. There is no known safe level of mercury and its disposal is governed by strict environmental guidelines.

There has been a 30-fold increase in the use of mercury in the industrialised world over the last 100 years.[35] It is present in low energy light bulbs, batteries, in some contact lens fluids and even some vaccines. Mercury can also be present in tuna fish and swordfish and, in some regions, drinking water.[36] Unfortunately there are myriad conditions associated with exposure to mercury. Mercury is highly toxic to human health[37] and is a powerful neurotoxin.[38] The greatest deposits of mercury tend to be found in the brain, kidneys and spinal cord neurological tissue, although the long list of affected organs also includes the gut, skin and the heart as well as the blood. Similarly, the symptoms associated with mercury poisoning are many and varied: chronic fatigue,[39] headaches,[40] depression,[41] memory loss,[41] autism,[42] attention deficit and hyperactivity disorder (ADHD),[43] autoimmune diseases,[44] diabetes, stomach pains, arthritis, infertility, asthma, insomnia, nervousness, anxiety…the list goes on.

Yet mercury accounts for half of every amalgam filling given to dental patients over the last 150 years. Why? Because amalgam fillings are long lasting, cheap and from a purely technical point of view are an ideal dental material. For years it was believed that the toxic properties of mercury were rendered inert when it was mixed with other metals that make up the other 50 per cent of an amalgam filling, namely tin, zinc, copper and silver. However, it is now well established that hot drinks, tobacco smoke and the process of chewing – especially gum – and even brushing our teeth release tiny amounts of mercury vapour from amalgam fillings. This is known as offgassing and can potentially lead to a chronic low-level poisoning that can affect people for decades.

Exactly why mercury is still used as a dental material is a contentious issue. The paradox is obvious: legislation exists to protect us from the harmful effects of incorrect disposal of mercury, yet dentists can install it onto our teeth with impunity. Some people in the dentistry profession argue that the risk of exposure only exists during the fitting and removal of amalgam fillings. Others point to the fact that mercury has never been tested for safety and that there is, therefore, no scientific proof that it is indeed safe to be used in the body.

Unfortunately, for two reasons, proof is very hard to establish. First, in the case of amalgam fillings, mercury is released in very small doses over a long period of time and people simply don't usually exhibit any immediate and noticeable side-effects. Second, it is associated with a huge range of disorders that are also caused by other factors. This almost always leads to mercury being overlooked as a culprit. Mercury has the ability to cross the blood brain barrier and adversely affect the central nervous system as well as being deposited in the brain. The amount of mercury in the brain has been found to be proportionate to the number of amalgam fillings in someone's mouth.[45]

Sweden, Norway and Denmark have legislated against mercury on environmental grounds and in the USA, crematoria are subject to strict guidelines, such is the danger to air quality of the burning of amalgam fillings.

Depending on their overall composition, the toxicity of mercury fillings, which can be measured with a mercury vapour analyser machine, varies. An example of a problematic scenario is when a person has a gold filling adjacent to an amalgam filling. The close proximity and mixture of these two metals combined with salt water in the saliva creates a virtual battery in the mouth, giving rise to a galvanic current (measured in micro-amps) and, consequently, a higher release of toxic mercury vapour. A common, but disturbing, clinical find is when a gold crown has been fitted on top of an existing amalgam filling which can, through the galvanic currents, hugely increase the rate of vapour being discharged. As we are discovering, mercury is by its very nature mercurial! Neither stable nor rendered inert nor contained in an amalgam, but instead leaching mercury vapour. We know that fillings leach mercury into the body and yet the World Health Organisation has stated that there is no safe level of mercury exposure.[46]

Mercury, like antibiotics, attacks microbes. When ingested, it leaks into the gut, compromising the gut flora and suppressing the healthy immune function and potentially contributing to autoimmune conditions.

The mercury level present in the umbilical cord blood supplying a newborn baby is in direct relation to the amount of amalgam fillings the mother has in her mouth.[47]

When inhaled, around 70 to 80 per cent of mercury vapour gets absorbed into the bloodstream with obvious implications for neurological health. We know that long-term inhalation of elemental mercury vapour may cause damage to the central nervous system, kidneys and stomach.[48]

Many people with healthy gut bacteria are able to break down mercury and remain somewhat free of the effects of exposure for years. However, over several decades, this ability can become compromised and the job of dealing with mercury passes to the liver, kidneys and the bladder. At this stage, traces of mercury can be present in the urine. These traces prevent the healing of a damaged or inflamed bladder wall. Of course, in a gut that is already compromised, as is regularly the case in people with PBS, the effects of mercury can be felt much sooner.

Clinical experience has shown that many people, upon learning of the effects of mercury poisoning, have had their amalgam fillings removed and have felt better as a result. This has also been confirmed by a German amalgam risk assessment study, which concluded:

> Removal of dental amalgam leads to permanent improvement of various chronic complaints in a relevant number of patients in various trials. Summing up, available data suggests that dental amalgam is an unsuitable material for medical, occupational and ecological reasons.[49]

It won't surprise you to learn that I often recommend the removal of amalgam fillings when appropriate.

WARNING

If you decide to have your amalgams removed it is imperative that it is undertaken gradually by a specialist mercury-free dentist who is familiar with keeping mercury vapour exposure to you, the patient, to a minimum. They should be replaced with suitable biocompatible non-metal material.

It is possible to measure the galvanic current of amalgam fillings and this often helps my patients make an informed decision as to which fillings are potentially discharging most mercury.

Once the teeth are completely clear of amalgam fillings it is possible to go on a mercury detox, details of which can be found in the Appendix. There's no guarantee that it will cure PBS, but, given the links between mercury and gut and kidney, replacing any amalgams you may have could play an important role in the managing of your symptoms. Not everyone who has PBS/IC necessarily has mercury fillings, but for those who have, I believe it is worth investigating the mercury levels you have. As I have mentioned, it is absolutely vital that the fillings are removed with impeccable attention to detail and safety as, just as I have encountered radical improvements from PBS after mercury removal, I have also come across those whose PBS began after the removal of their amalgams with lack of regard to its safety.

MERCURY, MADNESS AND MILLINERY

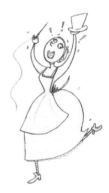

The term 'as mad as a hatter' originates from exposure to mercury in 19th century millinery. Working in often unventilated factories, hat makers of the 1800s used a mercury-based solution to mat the fibres of animal fur in the manufacture of top hats. After continually inhaling mercury vapour, many of these factory workers experienced trembling, loss of coordination, slurred speech, memory loss, fatigue and personality change. Making hats, it seemed, was a job that would drive you mad.

Mercury is no longer used in millinery but remains widespread in dentistry. It is not then surprising that there are studies that show dental personnel are more likely to have more problems with cognition,[50] produce less of the antioxidant glutathione[51] (a necessary ingredient for the detoxification pathways), and have an increased occurrence of neurological symptoms: psychosomatic symptoms, problems with memory, concentration, fatigue and sleep disturbance.[52]

Jane, age 44

Jane, a mother of three, had the classic PBS symptoms: frequent and urgent urination, occasional soreness of the urethra and a semi-constant bearing-down pain in the bladder area. She had a history of UTIs which had been treated with antibiotics. Her PBS pain was episodic and had been slowly getting worse for over a year.

Jane also had low energy and episodes of extreme fatigue, cold extremities, irritability, severe constipation, poor concentration and memory, hay fever every spring, a blocked nose most of the time and low libido and headaches.

After consulting master herbalist and acupuncturist Stephen Macallan, Jane took part in a series of tests. These revealed that she had Candida overgrowth, mercury poisoning, low stomach acid, numerous vitamin deficiencies and a poor ability to detoxify.

To combat the Candida, Jane began a regime of good quality probiotics, the anti-fungal capryllic complex, herbal tea (to cleanse and soothe the urinary tract) and a herbal aid (to improve bowel cleansing). The regime excluded sugar and yeast.

To help detoxification, Stephen recommended that Jane take a weekly far-infrared sauna.

In the month that followed the start of the regime, Jane enjoyed improved all-round general health including improved energy levels. Her urinary tract symptoms were marginally reduced and a little libido had returned, but sexual activity appeared to aggravate the cystitis symptoms. So for the following month, Jane's programme was augmented with a herbal heavy metal detox formula, resulting in an almost complete alleviation of pain.

There was still the mercury to deal with, however, and after her initial apprehension, Jane agreed to have her five amalgam fillings replaced. Within a a month all the pain disappeared. Occasionally the pain returned, but each time it was easier to bear as, over time, the cleansing and detoxing effect of the probiotic and a herbal tea regime continued to clear the mercury from her body.

After a year, Jane was completely clear of all her PBS symptoms.

Cavitations – dental infections

Another factor in dentistry and oral health that can have far-reaching effects on general health is the formation of cavitations. Cavitations occur where an area of jaw bone in the mouth dies, and becomes infected or decayed, usually due to a disruption of blood flow. During this process, the bone softens, becomes porous and changes in colour. Chronic inflammation then follows, forming a pus that seeps through into a sinus or other passage in the body. From here, the dead (necrotic) material can find its way into the rest of the body.

Because cavitations can exist deep within the jaw, they are often walled off from the surface by teeth, bridges and crowns and are commonly not picked up by x-rays. They can, however, in some instances be identified by a specialist Cavitat machine, a device for measuring bone density in the mouth and identifying possible pockets where poisonous bacteria could be building up, with the potential for leaking into the body.

Cavitations can be caused by dentistry as well as bacterial or toxic factors. These include procedures such as extractions, root canal work, injections, periodontal surgery and heat from drilling.

If a tooth is incorrectly pulled out, debris, in the form of broken periodontal ligaments which previously attached the tooth to the jaw, or fragments of extracted teeth, can be left behind if not thoroughly scraped out. These have the potential to decompose in the jaw and, though the jaw bone will heal, the infection from the debris can live on, creating the start of a cavitation.

After root canal treatment, which involves drilling into the nerve in order to kill it, dentists attempt to disinfect and kill off bacteria in the affected location. However, it is impossible to make the area completely sterile as bacteria can migrate into the body via microtubules, tiny rigid hollow tubes that lie deep in the root matrix.

Other causes of cavitations include dead or infected teeth, abscesses and cysts, periodontal disease, anaesthetic by-products and other dental materials and chemicals. A single cavitation in a healthy individual is unlikely to cause major health problems. The challenges arise where multiple cavitations exist, particularly in people with compromised immune systems. Cavitations have been linked with a wide range of disorders including:

- arthritis
- asthma
- bacterial endocarditis
- eczema
- neurological disorders
- tonsillitis.[53]

The spread of toxins throughout the body as a direct consequence of cavitations reduces the ability of the immune system to deal with chronic diseases such as PBS.

Cavitations can be either surgically removed or, if detected early, treated with therapies that assist the body's natural healing processes. The non-surgical options can also be used in conjunction with removal procedures to provide a holistic treatment plan. However, a long-standing and toxic cavitation usually has to be resolved surgically.

The link between conventional dentistry and compromised immune functionality is a controversial one: many orthodox dentists argue that there is no connection whatsoever, while some holistic dentists will reiterate that there is no such thing as a sterile root canal, and therefore in many cases the tooth will need to be extracted in order to lighten the immunological burden.

Cranial motion

Slightly less controversial these days is the subject of cranial motion. Cranial motion, also known as cranial rhythm, describes the process by which the bones in the head – and there are 27 of them – move in concert with one another.

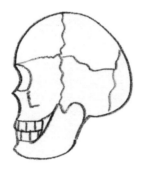

Up to the mid-20th century it was believed that, as we grew up, the bones in our head fused together to create a rigid structure. However, it is now accepted across all medical professions that not only do they remain separate, but that the oscillations between these bones play an important role in our health – and not just in the head itself.

If the cranial plates become jammed, cranial motion is blocked. And again, dental procedures can cause just such a blockage, with a whole range of unintended consequences in unexpected parts of the body. For example, a bridge crossing the maxillary mid-line (between the front two teeth) will fix the sutures, thus stopping cranial movement. This can affect the functioning of organs such as the bladder and the kidney, in turn compromising adrenal heath and the ability to urinate. Braces, crowns, dentures and other dental therapies can also fuse teeth together, affecting cranial movement and causing the onset of symptoms very quickly. As well as kidney and bladder problems, these can include depression, claustrophobia, irritability, facial pain, eye pain and mental confusion.[53]

In these instances, the only option is to make cuts in any bridges, crowns, and so on that are causing the blockage. This enables cranial movement to be re-established very quickly with a similarly rapid improvement in symptoms. Once the necessary dental work has been done it is then advisable to consult a cranial osteopath who is able to free up the potential blocks.

You can minimise the risk of all these oral hazards by opting to be treated by a holistic dentist who understands the science of cranial motions and the risks of amalgam fillings and cavitations.

CHAPTER 5

Painful Bladder Syndrome and Diet

As we have seen so far, diagnosing and treating PBS are far from straightforward. And the same is true when it comes to recommending a healthy diet for PBS patients. In fact, many so-called healthy foods have been shown to make symptoms worse for some people.

When it comes to diet, we are all unique in that each of us has our own set of individual tolerances and sensitivities to different types of food – and the quantities we can consume them in. Person A, for example, may consume a large portion of a known bladder irritant with no consequence whatsoever, while the mere trace of it may be sufficient to spark a flare-up in Person B. Another reason for this variability is that there are so many factors that cause the symptoms of pain, urgency and frequency in cases of PBS. This can make it difficult to isolate a single culprit.

It's unlikely then that a practitioner will tell you what you should and should not eat and drink to control your symptoms without understanding your unique circumstances first. However, there are foods and food types that most PBS patients agree are bad news. In alphabetical order these are:

- alcohol
- aspartame and artificial sweeteners

- carbonated drinks

- chocolate

- coffee and tea

- fruit (especially citrus, berries and pineapple)

- onions

- soy sauce

- spices, especially cooked chilli

- tomatoes

- vinegar.

Inflammation and diet

The modern western diet is a major factor in chronic inflammation. Many foods such as crisps, white bread, most breakfast cereals and other refined carbohydrates and sugars are known to have an overall inflammatory effect. An imbalance of omega 3 and omega 6 fats in the diet (something that has become increasingly common over the last 50 years) is also, in my clinical experience, likely to predispose a person to chronic inflammation.

As well as being good for health generally, a diet low on the glycaemic index (GI) is especially recommended if you have chronic inflammation. Low GI foods are those that release carbohydrates slowly, thus preventing spikes in blood sugar levels. A diet which predominates in high glycaemic foods results in increased inflammation in the body as a result of chronic hyperinsulinemia. The table below shows a simplified breakdown of the glycaemic index. Foods that are inflammatory for the body are often more processed and higher on the glycaemic index.

Table 5.1 Glycaemic index of foods

Low GI (55 or less)	Medium GI (56–59)	High GI (70 and above)
Most vegetables Legumes, pulses, beans Most whole grains Nuts Dairy Animal proteins	Brown rice Brown breads Quinoa Some fruits	Sugar, glucose, maltose, etc. Most breakfast cereals Refined grains such as white rice Carbonated drinks Crisps Pastries, cakes, white bread Some fruits

Even the good foods, however, are not ready-made for the fight against chronic inflammation. First, we have to extract from them the key ingredients that enable us to produce our weapons against inflammation: prostaglandins. Prostaglandins are derived from fatty acids and synthesised in the body where they have several roles, among them regulating our response to inflammation.

There are three types of prostaglandin, P1, P2 and P3. P2 is responsible for raising the immune response while P1 and P3, by dilating the blood vessels and reducing clotting, temper the painful effects of inflammation. Of course, under normal circumstances, both processes need to work together to fight infection, injury or viruses. However, in the case of chronic inflammation, where the immune response remains active long after the cause has been dealt with, the mechanisms of P2 need to be held in check.

Drugs have been developed to suppress the production of P2, and in turn, the pain and inflammation associated with ongoing immune responses. Though successful in this objective, they were also found to cause heart disease. This is why I believe that the best way to combat chronic inflammation is to find the right balance between inflammatory and anti-inflammatory foods in our diet and work to relieve other underlying causes. These include emotional stress and a lack of exercise as both of these factors make it difficult for the body to detoxify. Another major cause is tobacco smoking. Carcinogens in tobacco smoke known as nitrosamines are linked to chronic inflammation in the pancreas (pancreatitis) as well as pancreatic cancer and lung cancer.

For people with PBS, the symptoms of pain, urgency and frequency are the direct consequences of chronic inflammation of the bladder wall. So as well as avoiding foods that are irritating and inflammatory there are certain foods, antioxidants, herbs and therapies that can, as part of a holistic PBS treatment programme, reduce inflammation and by extension help manage the condition.

PBS and gluten intolerance

Many PBS patients also have coeliac disease or non-coeliac gluten intolerance. Coeliac disease, a genetic condition, is an immune reaction to gluten, a protein present in wheat, rye and barley. These foods are widely consumed as part of the standard western diet. I have seen many inflammatory and chronic conditions respond favourably to the exclusion of gluten from the diet. I have particularly noticed this with patients with PBS/IC. I am not the only one to observe this link. IC researcher Wendy Cohen also found there to be significant relief for many people after the exclusion of gluten from the diet.[54]

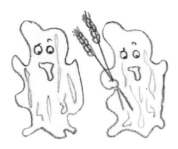

People with gluten intolerance, whether coeliac or otherwise, can experience a wide range of painful and distressing symptoms if they consume gluten – even in the smallest quantity for some. Those who also have PBS are likely to experience more intense PBS symptoms and more regular flare-ups. This is because gluten exacerbates almost any inflammatory condition, in particular leaky gut and 'leaky bladder'.

If you find that gluten is affecting you, and you've not been checked for coeliac disease, it's advisable to ask your doctor for the tests. If you have the condition, you will need to adopt a gluten-free diet. If, on the other hand, you don't have coeliac disease, you could try a process of elimination to identify which food is causing the PBS flare-up.

With almost every case of PBS I have treated, the removal of gluten from the patient's diet has dramatically reduced symptoms. I believe the link between the two is so convincing that I urge all my PBS patients, as a matter of course, to adopt a gluten-free diet and allow approximately six weeks for noticing any improvement.

Herbs and other supplements

I shall be discussing the role that herbs and other dietary supplements can play in relieving PBS symptoms in both the short and long term. As a practising herbalist, I have treated many PBS patients by fine-tuning a regime involving a combination of herbs specific to each individual. And, while I cannot claim to possess the elusive cure for PBS, I have seen patients enjoy a rapid, and in many cases permanent, cessation of symptoms after adopting a suitable dietary and herbal programme.

To help you understand the qualities and properties of the herbs and supplements most commonly used to treat PBS, Table 5.2 gives a handy guide that you can refer back to.

Table 5.2 Handy guide to herbs and supplements

Supplement	How it helps
Bromelain	Bromelain, an extract from the stem of the pineapple plant, has important anti-inflammatory properties. It has also been shown to prevent scar tissue, which, in PBS, reduces bladder capacity and causes swelling and pain elsewhere in the body. Best taken on an empty stomach, bromelain is commonly combined with the antihistamine quercitin (see below) by manufacturers of diet supplements.
Buchu (Agothosma betulina)	Indigenous to South Africa and containing strong antibacterial agents and essential oils, buchu is one of nature's best antiseptics. As well as reducing acidity in the body (it is a traditional remedy for gout, which is caused by raised levels of uric acid in the blood), it is particularly indicated if a woman is having clear/white vaginal discharges. It is also indicated and useful for non-bacterial prostatitis. The essential oils in the buchu leaf work on contact with the infection but can have a slightly irritating effect on the bladder and urinary tract. For this reason, I always advise my patients to use it in conjunction with marshmallow root (see below).

Cornsilk (Zea mays)	A mild diuretic and antiseptic, cornsilk reduces frequency and has the demulcent effect of soothing pain caused by bladder, urinary tract and urethral infections as well as prostate disorders. It has also been used for treating bed-wetting, obesity and premenstrual syndrome. As cornsilk is, literally, the silk from the corn cob, it is important to ensure the product you buy is organic and free of pesticides.
Cranberry	Cranberries have an anti-adhesion effect on the urinary tract. This can help to inhibit the escalation of existing UTIs and the development of new infection by preventing bacteria from adhering – and then multiplying – in the urinary tract. Cranberry also acts as a mild antiseptic, reduces allergic responses and helps to correct the pH (acid/alkali) balance in urine. For those wanting to try cranberries, it is best to use a solid extract, available in capsules or pills, or make your own juice by soaking cranberries in water, blending them and making your own version of the juice. Many commercial juices contain copious amounts of sugar or, even worse, artificial sweeteners or corn syrup. However, cranberry is not the panacea for all urinary ills: it can be useful for those who have a tendency to UTIs, but for those with PBS it can actually make the situation worse. Many have a reaction with cranberries, with a severity similar to that of coffee.
D-mannose	A naturally occurring substance, which can be very useful in treating urinary tract infections. It stops the adherence of E. coli to the urinary tract.[55]

cont.

Table 5.2 Handy guide to herbs and supplements *cont.*

Supplement	How it helps
Fennel seeds (Foeniculum vulgare)	Used in many traditions of ancient medicine. The seeds are slightly diuretic and are enormously soothing for the urinary system and digestive system. They can be helpful to encourage healthy menstruation and are antispasmodic, so great for cramps and spasms.
Glucosamine sulphate and chondroitin sulphate	Glucosamine helps to restore the glycoaminoglycan (GAG) layer. It is useful as part of a whole-person approach to repair the bladder lining.[56] Chondroitin has also been shown to be useful for those with PBS as it, too, is used by the body for epithelial integrity of the mucous layer of both gut and bladder. It is usually worth taking a supplement that combines both together.
Gokshura (Tribulas terrestris semen)	Gokshura is an Ayurvedic medicine used in the treatment of a wide variety of disorders. It is also known as 'puncture vine'. Its value to PBS patients lies in its rejuvenative and replenishing effects on the urinary tract and bladder. It contains anti-infection constituents and has an anti-inflammatory effect on the urinary tract. Gokshura can act like a mild antihistamine and is linked to promoting emotional and mental wellbeing. It enhances the body's ability to produce the adrenal hormone DHEA. It also has a hormonal balancing effect for women.

L-arginine	Believed to increase blood flow to the bladder, L-arginine is one of the amino acids that make up the proteins in our food. Findings from research carried out at Yale University in 1996[57] suggest that L-arginine can help reduce the symptoms of pain and frequency in some PBS patients. However, some patients have found an exacerbation of symptoms with taking this amino acid.
Liquorice (Glycyrrhiza glabra radix)	This is a strong adrenal and urinary tract restorative. It can be used to encourage the body to restore adrenal hormones such as cortisol. It is a specific herb to be used with 'burn out' and has an anti-inflammatory effect on the urinary tract and encourages healthy production of mucous and the epithelial layers and encourages liver detoxification pathways. It has ulcer healing properties.

(It is contraindicated in those with high blood pressure. If someone is taking liquorice medicinally then blood pressure should be regularly monitored as over periods of four to six weeks it can cause retention of salt and hypokalaemia. However, your practitioner will monitor your blood pressure whilst taking it.) |
| Lotus seeds (Nelumo nucifera semen) | These are useful for their ability to help with urinary incontinence and for their ability to nourish mucous membranes in the digestive system, and can be used for their restorative effect on the bladder wall. They can be eaten as a food and can be briefly dry fried and added into food or soup. |

cont.

Table 5.2 Handy guide to herbs and supplements *cont.*

Supplement	How it helps
Marshmallow root (Althea officinalis)	Containing pain-relieving polysaccharides and the mild diuretic, asparagin (also present in asparagus), marshmallow root helps the body excrete bacteria associated with cystitis while soothing the burning pain that may be experienced. Its anti-inflammatory constituencies also help with gastro-intestinal and urinary tract infections and the repair of inflamed mucous membranes.
Prelief®	This over-the-counter product is, essentially, calcium glycerophosphate, which neutralises acidic foods by raising their pH. It is designed to enable people intolerant to high acidy to eat foods that would otherwise be excluded from their diets. As its name suggests, Prelief®, which is available in tablet or powder form, needs to be taken with a meal. My concern regarding this is that it encourages the ingestion of food which contains constituents that the body doesn't want. Also, prolonged use could have a detrimental effect on acid levels in the stomach. I would recommend that this is used in an emergency, but not necessarily as part of therapeutic regime.
Pumpkin seeds	The anti-inflammatory properties of pumpkin seeds are well established, having first been explored by native Americans in the treatment of kidney, bladder and intestinal disorders. More recently, research has shown that they can improve the flow of urine through the bladder and urethra and reduce the risk of developing prostate inflammation.

Purnanava/ Indian hogweed (Boerhaavia diffusa radix)	This is known in Ayurveda to encourage and support healthy kidney function. It is usually combined with other herbs such as gokshura to support urinary health.
Quercitin	Quercitin is a natural antihistamine and also has anti-inflammatory and antioxidant effects. Shown to significantly reduce symptoms associated with chronic prostatitis, quercitin can also improve conditions such as hay fever, asthma and upper respiratory tract infections.

Many patients notice positive effects from taking this supplement. This has also been demonstrated by a medical trial, which found that it was 'well tolerated and provided significant symptomatic improvement in patients with PBS'.[58]

Often paired with bromelain (see above). |
| Sea buckthorn (Hippophae L.) | First used in Tibet over 1000 years ago, sea buckthorn is still widely used today by herbalists to strengthen the mucous membranes in the urogenital tract. It has been shown to be highly effective in treating women with partial cervix erosion and vaginal inflammation, due in no small part to its high values of vitamin E and natural carotenoids. Other names for sea buckthorn include sandthorn, sallowthorn and seaberry. |

cont.

Table 5.2 Handy guide to herbs and supplements *cont.*

Supplement	How it helps
Shilajit	This is a mineral which is made from fossilised vegetable matter and is an exudate that seeps out of the rocks in the Himalayas. The raw ingredient needs to be correctly processed according to ancient Ayurvedic processes. It is reputed to act as a strong adaptagen and general tonic. It is a mineral medicine, which has a strong rejuvenative effect on the kidneys and bladder. It contains humic acid, which helps the absorption of minerals into the tissues and cells. I have found it of enormous value in PBS, especially when someone is relatively stable, as a way of preventing further flare-ups and to encourage remission.
Turmeric (Curcuma longa)	The therapeutic benefits of turmeric are many and varied, and can be felt by people with conditions ranging from rheumatoid arthritis to stomach ulcers. A powerful antioxidant, turmeric, which contains the active constituent curcumin, also reduces inflammation and histamine levels and promotes liver detoxification and improved circulation.
Uva ursi (Arctostaphylos uva-ursi)	Also known as bearberry or kinnikinnick, uva ursi has a strong antiseptic effect, particularly in the urinary tract, bladder and kidneys. It can help with acute yeast infections such as Candida albicans by reducing acidity in the body. For this reason, uva ursi is also good for symptoms involving heat or burning during urination. It also contains potent essential oils and should be taken with marshmallow root and/or cornsilk.

Varuna (Crataeva nurvula)	Native to India and Bangladesh, varuna is a traditional Ayurvedic herb used commonly for treating problems in the kidney, prostate and urinary tract. A chemical in varuna called lupeol inhibits inflammation, while the herb also forms a soothing film over the mucous membrane (known as a demulcent) which reduces pain when urinating. Varuna is also known as barun and three-leaved caper.
Vitamin A (Retinol or beta carotene)	Vitamin A plays an important role in the repair of mucous membranes in the gut, bladder and urinary tract. An oxidant, it helps to protect against disease and promote cell growth. Available in tablet and capsule form in health food shops and supermarkets, vitamin A is present in many foods such as fish, eggs, milk and butter as well as dark green and orange vegetables.

BUT BEFORE YOU START...

Although you can buy the herbs and supplements listed here at health food shops, supermarkets or online stores, I strongly recommend that you discuss your case with a qualified herbalist before starting any herb-based regime. Herbs and supplements can be contraindicated in pregnancy or while breastfeeding, with certain medical conditions such as a heart condition or high blood pressure, with certain medical drugs, as well as in other situations. For example, some herbs can render the contraceptive pill less effective, or make other medications more powerful. PBS is a multi-faceted and complex condition and every patient has different symptoms, varying levels of tolerance to diet supplements and, in some cases, side-effects. The most effective herbal programme you can get is one that is designed specifically for you, your symptoms and your personal circumstances.

That said, I also believe that a natural approach to a long-term condition such as PBS is infinitely preferable to conventional pain relievers and antibiotics because:

- antibiotics kill good bacteria in our body as well as bad, so we always pay a price for the benefit they provide. They are mostly ineffective for cases of PBS/IC. Other medications targeting PBS are often only helpful when taking them, rather than having a restorative effect on the body, and can produce distressing side-effects in some people.

- over extended periods, we develop immunities to prescription drugs and painkillers. This usually leads to increased dosages, resulting in the increased intensity of side-effects and even more good bacteria in our bodies being killed off.

Another complication with long-term reliance on medication is that UTIs are becoming increasingly resistant to antibiotics. One reason for this is their overuse in modern farming methods, leading to the introduction of antibiotic-resistant bacteria in the human gut.[59]

A recent study in Hong Kong,[60] for example, found that farm animals carry a gene which can activate resistance to gentacimin, an antibiotic commonly used to treat UTIs. When we eat the meat of these animals, the resistant gene can find its way to our gut and hamper efforts to treat infections.

As well as providing good reason to opt for a natural treatment plan for PBS, studies like this also reinforce the case for organically produced foods.

Summary

Before we move on to Part II, where we'll be looking at diet and other strategies to manage PBS, let's briefly summarise the key points so far.

PBS is a chronic condition in which the bladder wall becomes inflamed, causing bladder pain, increased frequency and urinary urgency.

PBS flare-ups are episodes when the symptoms intensify. Flare-ups vary in severity and duration from patient to patient.

Cystitis and UTIs are distinct from PBS. They are caused by infection in the bladder and urinary tract as opposed to inflammation and damage to the bladder wall. UTIs come on suddenly, are usually short-lived and respond to antibiotics and natural treatments. PBS is a chronic condition and does not usually respond to antibiotics.

Diagnosing PBS is problematic. Patients are often misdiagnosed and treated for a range of unrelated conditions with similar symptoms over extended periods with no improvement. It's important to rule out cancers in the urinary tract and the bladder as part of a thorough diagnosis with your doctor or urologist. Other conditions to check for include overactive bladder, haemorrhagic cystitis and chronic prostatitis.

PBS frequently coexists with other disorders such as:

- autoimmune problems (e.g. systemic lupus erythematosus [SLE], where the immune system mistakenly attacks its own healthy body tissue)
- pelvic problems, including pelvic floor dysfunction
- vulvodynia – chronic pain in the vulva
- fibromyalgia – a painful musculoskeletal disorder
- chronic fatigue syndrome
- food allergies such as coeliac disease
- panic attacks and anxiety.

Conventional treatment for PBS usually revolves around drugs to relieve pain, frequency and urgency, inflammation relief and the use of intravesical therapies to repair the bladder wall.

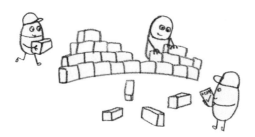

Holistic treatments for PBS focus on protecting the bladder wall by optimising the health of all organs through which toxins and irritants can develop and find their way to the bladder. Methods include:

- identifying food intolerances and allergies
- rebalancing the bacterial flora in the gut to combat yeast overgrowth and pH imbalances

- tackling blocked liver detoxification pathways and adrenal fatigue

- protecting the psoas muscle from over-frequent contractions and releasing stress from the body

- identifying toxins and physical stress factors resulting from dentistry such as mercury fillings, cavitations and blocked cranial motion

- encouraging the healing of the bladder lining through the use of herbs and nutrients.

PART II

Managing Painful Bladder Syndrome

CHAPTER 6

Diet and the Gut

As the core of our whole system, the gut is central to any holistic treatment programme for PBS. And how healthy the gut is depends on how it reacts to what we put inside it – in other words, how it copes with the food and drink we consume. Diet, then, is a probably the single most important element in your PBS management plan.

People with PBS almost always have leaky gut as well. However, your practitioner can determine this through a gut permeability test. A leaky gut allows toxins and bad bacteria to penetrate through its tight junctions – the gateways through which only nutrients are meant to enter our bloodstream.

As I have discussed, a large factor in ongoing leaky gut is the consumption of foods that your body is intolerant to. It is through these intolerances that people experience the pain and discomfort of PBS and, in particular, PBS flare-ups. For this reason, a three-stage dietary adjustment process will help you to, first, alleviate the symptoms, second, prevent further damage to the gut and, third, make a start on restoring gut and bladder health.

Stage 1: Alleviating PBS symptoms
Singling out exactly which foods are aggravating your bladder and contributing to PBS symptoms is a process of

trial and error. Each person will react differently to different irritants; however, as we saw earlier, the usual suspects are:

- alcohol
- aspartame and artificial sweeteners
- carbonated drinks
- chocolate
- coffee and tea
- fruit (especially citrus, berries and pineapple)
- onions
- soy sauce
- spices, especially cooked chilli
- tomatoes
- vinegar.

Use this list as a starting point and experiment by consuming one item at a time for a few days. You may find that removing high-acid foods makes no difference at all, while cutting out caffeine by avoiding tea, coffee and chocolate coincides with a noticeable reduction in PBS symptoms. It's also important to consider that sometimes a food will react within a few hours, whilst others might take 24 hours.

Once we have identified exactly which foods and drinks are causing an initial irritating effect on your bladder then they can be removed from the diet. While this is not a cure, cutting out dietary triggers will relieve the worst of your symptoms and reduce the frequency and intensity of PBS flare-ups. We can also now work towards stopping the flow of toxins through the gut wall to the bladder.

Stage 2: Preventing further damage to the gut and bladder wall

This stage involves further experimentation with diet as we seek to establish which foods not only penetrate a leaky gut, but cause the gut to become permeable in the first place. Many of the foods in the list above are culprits here too; however, the classic causes are gluten, soya and sugar. Before you read the full list and condemn yourself to a life of starvation, though, bear in mind that removing these foods is only a temporary measure – not a life sentence. Once your symptoms are under control, you can gradually try reintroducing the foods you miss most back into your diet and, in the process, isolate only those that are the causes of distress. And though the list does appear long, rest assured you still have plenty of options.

So, as we seek to narrow down the causes of leaky gut in your specific case, here are the foods to target:

- *Gluten*: top of the list, as almost everyone with PBS is gluten intolerant. Gluten can permeate the tight junctions of the small intestine, create inflammation and lead to immune reactions that aggravate leaky gut. Gluten is present in wheat, grains and processed food products that contain flour, so make sure you check the ingredients, as it is commonly in:

  o   wheat, barley, rye and oatmeal

  o   bread, scones, rolls, bagels and breaded ham

  o   pizza dough

  o   pretzels, biscuits and crispbreads, shortbread

  o   breakfast cereals, all bran, muesli

  o   cheap chocolate and drinking chocolate

  o   soups

- pate, meat and fish pastes
- luncheon meat
- sausages and burgers
- couscous
- pastry
- durum wheat pasta
- Yorkshire puddings, batter and pancakes
- stuffing
- crisps (those that contain wheat flour)
- gravy powder and cubes
- dumplings and shredded suet
- sauces, salad dressings, mustards
- chutneys and pickles
- malt vinegar
- semolina
- cakes, sponge puddings, cheesecakes, muffins.

It's a long list, yet by no means exhaustive – check food labels carefully when shopping. Many major supermarkets today have sections dedicated to foods that are free from gluten, wheat and dairy.

So to reiterate, you start by cutting out foods that cause you to experience a direct worsening of symptoms. It may not be possible to be completely symptom-free, but at least you have identified foods that are aggravating. Then it is usually worth cutting out gluten.

It is usually worth adjusting to the diet, making sure you are able to eat delicious alternatives and get used to eating in a different way. It might be that you notice a reduction in overall symptoms and feel better within yourself, which is a common experience. Then it is on to the next stage – clearing yeast overgrowth and correcting dysbiosis. Avoid the following:

- *Sugar:* anything ending in ose – such as maltose, dextrose, lactose, sucrose, fructose, glycerine, mannitol and sorbitol. This exclusion also includes maple syrup, golden syrup, molasses, rice syrup, date sugar and, of course, regular sugar.

- *Fruit juices:* all types including canned, bottled or frozen and smoothies. They are all high in sugar (see above).

- *Soya:* like gluten, soya can permeate the tight junctions of the small intestine and intensify PBS symptoms.

- *Coffee and tea:* avoid them absolutely.

- *Alcohol:* this hampers liver detoxification and increases the toxins in your gut.

- *Dairy:* milk, yoghurt and cheese (butter is usually okay).

- *Yeast:* including brewer's yeast, baker's yeast and any vitamin and mineral supplements that contain yeast. However, foods that contain yeast include:
  - most breads, rolls and crackers
  - beer and wine
  - sauerkraut vinegars
  - soy sauce
  - Worcestershire sauce
  - pickles and relishes.

- *Fresh and dried fruit*: for the first two to four weeks while yeast is brought under control. You should be able to reintroduce fruit to your diet after a month or so.

- *Peanuts and products that contain them*: they're potentially high in carcinogenic mould.

- *Pickled, smoked or dried meat, fish or poultry*.

Making it manageable

Clearly, to eliminate all these foods in one fell swoop from a typical diet is a big ask. And, of course, we are all different in what foods affect us as individuals. It's unlikely that every food listed above will affect you personally, so the challenge is to separate those that you can tolerate from those that you can't:

- *Step 1*: Identify and eliminate the most aggravating foods (e.g. you may personally find it is coffee, tea, tomatoes and alcohol).

- *Step 2*: Cut out gluten and give yourself a few weeks to get used to your diet and monitor your symptoms.

- *Step 3*: Avoid dairy (except butter), sugar and yeast whilst correcting the yeast and bacteria balance in the gut and starting the gut repair (see stage 3 on page 105).

Remember, the whole point is about restoring function and getting to a point of being able, once symptoms are controlled, to eat a wide and varied anti-inflammatory and nutrient-dense diet.

Keeping your diet gluten-free is almost always beneficial at this stage, but don't despair – it's not necessarily permanent. Once damage is repaired you can normally return to many of your favourite foods (unless you are diagnosed with coeliac disease or gluten intolerance).

This stage will take around three months to have any noticeable effects; you'll need a bit of willpower but the results are well worth it.

The gluten-free diet – what you can eat

At first glance, the list of foods that contain gluten may make you wonder if you'll ever eat again. There's no need to despair, however: meat-eaters and vegetarians alike on a gluten-free diet still have plenty of options. In their natural, unprocessed form, all these foods are gluten-free:

- amaranth

- arrowroot

- beans

- buckwheat

- corn and cornmeal

- eggs

- flax

- fresh fish

- fresh meat

- fresh poultry

- fruit and vegetables

- millet

- most dairy products (except those listed as excluded above)

- nuts

- quinoa

- rice

- seeds

- sorghum

- tapioca.

Other foods that are available in gluten-free form (always check the label) include:

- biscuits and crackers

- bread

- cereals

- chips

- croutons

- gravy

- pasta made from rice or vegetables

- soups and soup bases.

Stage 3: Restoring gut and bladder health

With your PBS flare-ups under control and a diet that excludes foods that were damaging your gut wall, we can start to restore the balance in the gut flora and the glycosaminoglycan (GAG) layer in the bladder.

It's a good idea to add plenty of (gluten-free) anti-inflammatory foods into your diet at this stage to maintain gut and bladder health. Examples of these include broccoli, cauliflower, sweet potatoes, spinach, turmeric, ginger, wild salmon, cod, mackerel, sardines, shiitake mushrooms.

Also highly beneficial are bone broths. Bone broths are widely used in many cultures. They are easy to make at home and can either be consumed as a stand-alone drink or used as a base for savoury rice dishes, soups or sauces. Because they are rich in a wide range of minerals, bone broths help to restore a leaky gut and bladder. They are rich in collagen, cartilage and glycosaminoglycans as well as minerals. Bones recommended are from chicken, fish and lamb, but it is totally necessary to be organic. Pork and beef are not usually recommended as they tend to be inflammatory in nature.

See the Appendix for how to prepare the bone broth. Depending on the bones you use, your bone broth will give you a whole range of minerals and nutrients, including:

- calcium
- phosphorous
- magnesium
- potassium
- sulphate
- fluoride
- collagen
- chondroitin
- glycine
- zinc.

Always make your broth at home as the commercially available products invariably contain monosodium glutamate (MSG) and high levels of salt.

As well as re-mineralising the body it is very helpful for restoring and healing the tight junctions of the gut and helping the immune system. The natural collagen and chondroitin are restorative for the bladder lining and for reducing inflammation.

Dysbiosis programme

It will usually be necessary to take antifungal and microbial herbs in order to rebalance the gut flora. Your practitioner will normally give you a number of antifungals to try for a few days, to ensure that there isn't any reaction. Usually five days is sufficient to know if the treatment is going to aggravate your bladder. If you can tolerate it, then usually it is suitable to take for a month. There are many dysbiosis medicines available. These are the ones I commonly recommend:

- *Myrrh (Commiphora molmol)*: a tree resin containing medicinal volatile oils, myrrh is a great healer and an antimicrobial and anti-inflammatory, boosting the number of white blood cells.

- *Caprylic acid*: promotes good bacteria in the gut, but avoid it if you have an inflammatory condition such as colitis. Although this is an acid I have found that it is usually well tolerated.

- *Grapefruit seed extract*: one of the best antifungal and antimicrobial agents, grapefruit seed extract has antiparasitic qualities and works well with caprylic acid in the form of caprylic complex. The capsule form is best for tackling yeast in the gut. Do not take with warfarin.

- *Horopito (Pseudowintera colorata) and aniseed*: a traditional Maori remedy for digestive complaints, combines well with aniseed to produce a synergistic effect that is highly antifungal and well tolerated in an inflamed gut.

- *Oregano (Origanum vulgare)*: not just a tasty cooking herb, oregano has many antibacterial and antifungal qualities. Also works well with grapefruit seed extract.

Using a number of medicines that accelerate healing in the gut, you can create a dysbiosis programme which will complement your new diet. Try this typical programme as part of your new regime:

WEEKS ONE TO FOUR
Begin taking antifungals such as myrrh and probiotics (see below) in capsule form:

- Myrrh: two capsules before breakfast; two capsules before evening meal.

- Probiotics: two capsules after breakfast; two capsules after evening meal.

Continue for one month.

WEEKS FIVE TO EIGHT
Replace myrrh with caprylic complex to prevent any Candida in the gut developing a resistance:

- Caprylic complex: two capsules before breakfast; two capsules before evening meal.

- Maintain the dosage of probiotics as usual.

Along with the gluten-free diet, this programme will help to restore balance in the gut and bring yeast overgrowth under control in around three months. It also improves general health and regulates bowel movements.

Probiotics

The consumption of beneficial bacteria or 'probiotics' is important for people with abnormal gut flora. Many fermented foods such as sauerkraut, salami and table olives provide a rich source of probiotics, but in western countries they are mainly taken in the form of supplements.

The practice of fermenting foods in eastern European, Asian and African cultures goes back many thousands of years. However, it wasn't until a Russian scientist, Ilya Ilyich

Metchnikoff (1845–1916), studied probiotics in detail that they began to be taken seriously as a viable treatment option.

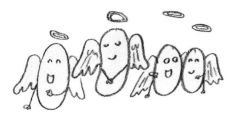

Metchnikoff discovered a link between the fermented milk products and the long and healthy lives enjoyed by Bulgarian country people and attributed this to a bacterium which he named Bulgarian bacillus. This became popular in western countries and Lactobacillis bulgaricus, as it is known today, is still prevalent in many yoghurt-based products.

The arrival of antibiotics somewhat overshadowed probiotics but research into their benefits continued long after Metchnikoff's death. While many Russian, Scandinavian and Japanese patients have been treated with probiotics for decades, their use in western countries was restricted mainly to farm animals. In recent years, however, the pendulum has swung back in their favour in this country and the use and popularity of probiotics are, once again, on the rise.

Probiotics have been known to improve – and in many cases cure – a wide range of conditions, many of which are beyond the scope of this book. So, in the following pages, I shall examine the families of bacteria that, in probiotic form, are most likely to benefit you as a PBS patient.

Lactobacilli

(Most common species: *L. acidophilus, L. bulgaricus, L. rhamnosus, L. plantarum, L. salivarius, L. reuteri, L. johnsonii, L. casei* and *L. delbrueckii*)

Lactobacilli bacteria reside in the gut, vagina and genital area and the mucous membranes of the mouth, throat, nose and upper respiratory tract. They also outnumber all other bacteria in the stomach and intestines where they form the mainstay of the defence against infection. Present in human breast milk, lactobacilli help to colonise the immune system in newborn babies. They produce lactic acid, which maintains the required acidity levels (pH 5.5–5.6) on mucous membranes so they can suppress the growth of pathogenic microbes. Lactobacilli also produce the antiseptic hydrogen peroxide and other antibacterial, antiviral and antifungal agents which prevent bad bacteria getting out of hand in the gut. They stimulate activity of neutrophils and macrophages, enable the synthesis of immunoglobins and are involved in cell renewal.

Bifidobacteria

(Most common species: *B. bifidum, B. breve, B. longum, B. infantis*)

The greatest concentrations of bifidobacteria are in the bowel, lower intestines, vagina and genital area, where they do much to promote good health. As well as protecting the gut from pathogens, bifidobacteria engage the immune system and provide nourishment for the body. Bifidobacteria synthesise amino acids, proteins and organic acids, not to mention a whole host of vitamins including:

- vitamin B1 (thiamin)

- vitamin B2 (riboflavin)

- vitamin B5 (pantothenic acid)

- vitamin B6 (pyridoxine)

- vitamin B12 (cobalamin)

- vitamin B13 (niacin)

- vitamin D (folic acid)

- vitamin K (phytomenadione).

Bifidobacteria also assist the absorption of calcium and iron.

Saccharomyces boulardii

This is a yeast from an extract of lychee fruit. In 1920, the French scientist, H. Boulard, learned that the extract was commonly used in China to treat diarrhoea. Three years later, he isolated the tropical strain of yeast in the extract, giving it the name Saccharomyces boulardii. Although still popular as an effective supplement for treating diarrhoea in children and adults, Saccharomyces boulardii could also be a powerful probiotic for combating Candida albicans.

Escherichia coli (E. coli)

E. coli comes in two types of strain – pathogenic (bad), which can cause serious illness, and physiological (good), which are an important part of healthy gut flora. Physiological E. coli strains are specific to the bowel and lower parts of the intestines and their appearance elsewhere, for example in the mouth, stomach or duodenum, is a sign of gut dysbiosis. The functions of physiological E. coli include digesting lactose and producing the B group of vitamins and vitamin K. They also produce amino acids and antibiotic-like substances called colicins and stimulate local and systemic immunity. One of the best defences against pathogenic E. coli strains is a healthy coating of their physiological siblings in the bowel and lower intestine.

Enterococcus faecium or Streptococcus faecalis

Isolated from stools, Enterococcus faecium or Streptococcus faecalis reside predominantly in the bowel where they break down proteins and ferment carbohydrates. They also fight pathogens by producing the antiseptic hydrogen peroxide and regulate acidity at pH 5.5.

Bacillus subtilis or soil bacteria

(Other species include: *B. licheniformis, B. cereus, B. brevis, B. mesentericus, B. pumilis*)

Soil bacteria were first discovered by German microbiologists looking for ways to treat soldiers with dysentery and typhoid during the Second World War. In the years following the war, studies into this probiotic intensified, with research facilities being set up in Russia, Italy, Finland, eastern Europe, China and Vietnam. This new, widespread attention led to the discovery of new species of soil bacteria, many of which were found to benefit animals and humans. Soil bacteria are spore-forming microbes which are unaffected by stomach acid, temperature change and most antibiotics and help to stimulate the immune systems. They have proved especially effective in the treatment of allergies and autoimmune disorders, but perhaps their greatest value lies in their ability to break down rotting matter and clear the way for new healthy flora to establish themselves. Soil bacteria also produce digestive enzymes as well as antiviral, antifungal and antibacterial substances.

Unlike most other probiotics, soil bacteria do not occur naturally in our body, nor do they colonise the gut. For this reason they are known as transitional bacteria as they provide their benefits as they pass through.

It is thought that our need for soil bacteria harks back to the period when our ancestors drank their water from wells and streams and their digestive systems learned to make good use of the natural substances it contained.[61]

The problem with commercially available probiotics

Most probiotics sold commercially are unlikely to be strong enough to treat a clinically diagnosed condition. In fact, many do not even provide the dosage they claim on the packaging, nor do they provide the wide variety of different bacteria necessary to repopulate a gut compromised by dysbiosis. To treat the type of gut abnormalities that usually accompany PBS, you are likely to need a blend of clinical-strength probiotics. Also, as all cases of PBS are unique in their associated disorders and, therefore, your symptoms, it's always best to consult a qualified practitioner who can advise you on the combination, dosage and course duration appropriate to your specific circumstances.

When you start using effective probiotics, you may experience tiredness, feel slightly nauseous or develop a rash on your skin. These symptoms are perfectly normal and are part of the 'die-off reaction'. The die-off reaction is the body's way of dealing with toxins being released by the dying viruses, bacteria and fungi. This is proof that your probiotics are working and the symptoms should disappear after a few days – or a few weeks at the most. If they persist longer than this, ask your practitioner to adjust your dosage.

Repairing the leaky gut

After carrying out two months of the dysbiosis programme following a strict no-sugar diet and taking well-tolerated antifungals and dysbiosis remedies and probiotics, most people are ready to move on to the leaky gut remedies.

It is essential to be taking probiotics throughout. However, there are a number of measures to restore the epithelial lining.

Butyric acid: This is available as a supplement and it is usually recommended that you take it for three to six months. A usual dose is one capsule three times daily. It is the essential ingredient that the body needs to repair the tight junctions and restore the gut mucosa and epithelium. This is of course only useful if you can tolerate it – it is contraindicated for those with ulceration of the bowel, such as colitis. Other sources of butyric acid are butter and ghee (see the recipe in the Appendix) and usually I recommend the liberal use of these in the diet.

L-glutamine: If you can't tolerate butyric acid then this is the next best alternative. It is another fuel necessary for the cells within the gut lining to repair and renew itself. It is available as a powder with the usual dosage being 5ml three times daily for a period of two to three months.

Bone soup: This can be an important part of re-mineralising the body and giving the necessary ingredients to restore the GAG layer in the bladder. If you are vegetarian then you will need to use my alternative broth (see the recipe in the Appendix).

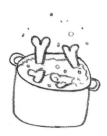

Butter or ghee: Saturated fat is essential for the repairing process. Organic butter is an excellent source, although in Ayurveda ghee is seen to be the ideal healing substance.

Ghee is cow's butter with the milk solids and water content removed and is a very pure food. It aids digestion, strengthens the body, increases energy levels, improves memory and brain functioning and increases longevity.

This is due to its chemical makeup – predominantly short-chain fatty acids which are easily absorbed, assimilated and metabolised by the body for energy release. Ghee is high in antioxidants (free radical scavengers). It also contains linoleic acid, a chemical that may have anti-carcinogenic properties, as well as vitamins A, D, E and K. Taking between 1 teaspoon and 2 tablespoons daily is usually recommended, in order to exploit its healing potential. A recipe for ghee can be found in the Appendix.

CHAPTER 7

Detoxification

Toxins, both internal and external, are at the root of many short- and long-term health problems. Through the foods we eat, the air we breathe, the medication we are prescribed and the lifestyles we live, we are exposed almost constantly to substances our bodies were never designed to encounter. That said, most people can repair the damage caused to their immune systems by toxins and, through detoxification strategies, remove them from the body.

Toxins – that is, substances that are harmful or hazardous to the human body – originate from an endless list of sources. Contrary to popular belief, they didn't first arrive along with manufacturing processes. People have been exposed to toxins for thousands of years through plants, weather conditions, emotional trauma and stress. Through adaptation we have developed effective defences against these types of toxin. The relatively recent revolution in industrialisation and modern farming techniques has, however, made our toxic burden a whole lot worse. Since the Second World War, more than two million new substances have been created and, in evolutionary terms at least, the human system is struggling to keep up: because we don't recognise these substances, we have no inbuilt defence against them.

The enemy within – and without

There are two types of toxin – internal and external. Internal toxins, or metabolic waste, are created as a by-product of the normal healthy functioning of the body. Ordinarily we are able to deal with and process them; however, if our detoxification pathways are compromised in some way and not adequately able to process toxins generated by the body, or are exposed to environmental toxins, our body can store them in fat cells and cell membranes. Unless we actively encourage detoxification, the toxic load will increase until the body can no longer cope, resulting in some breakdown of health. External toxins are created outside the human body and are a fact of daily life. To list just a few, we expose ourselves to external toxins when we:

- shower, bathe, wash our hair or shave: through the toiletries we use

- clean our homes: through cleaning products such as detergents and polishes

- eat non-organic foods: through the pesticides used in their production.

Workplaces can also be toxic. While workers such as factory operatives, mechanics and painters and decorators are especially exposed, even office workers don't escape external toxins: they can be found in computers, printers and photocopiers, not to mention the heady mix of personal hygiene products of large numbers of people in relatively small, confined spaces.

Getting it out of the system

Detoxification, then, is a good idea for all of us, whatever our underlying health. For people with PBS, however, cleansing the body of unwanted chemicals forms a central part of the recovery plan. This is because people with PBS are particularly sensitive to toxins as they get through a compromised gut wall and aggravate an already vulnerable bladder wall. Other effects experienced by people sensitive to toxins include reduced immunity, autoimmune diseases and muscle pain, all of which I find frequently coexisting in people with PBS.

Detoxification is the process of rendering toxic substances harmless and then excreting them, something our bodies do naturally every day. Problems arise, however, when a person's capability to detoxify is compromised or the type and/or quantity of toxins causes an unmanageable workload. In this scenario, the intoxicated organs and tissues in the body remain uncleansed and an imbalance occurs. This is when we need to follow a detoxification programme.

In the book *Natural Detoxification*,[62] the build-up of toxins is likened to the accumulation of water in a water butt (rainbarrel), as in the extract in the box below.

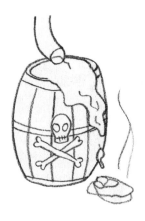

THE RAINBARREL EFFECT

People are subjected to a wide range of physical, emotional and environmental stresses that contribute to their toxic burden. The body burden can be viewed as 'rain', which gradually fills the 'rainbarrel' of our bodies. We can adjust to a few stressors, but as the rainbarrel level rises, our metabolism loses its adaptability and we begin to experience toxic overload. Our detoxification mechanisms no longer function adequately and the body cannot maintain its balance. We develop symptoms because our toxin levels are too high. Eventually, the body cannot cope with its toxic burden and our rainbarrel overflows, resulting in disease.

If we periodically empty our rainbarrel with detoxification procedures, we can withstand the stresses of moderate exposures. However, if our rainbarrel continues to fill, additional stressors will cause it to overflow, with resulting symptoms. This is why some exposures can cause us distressing symptoms, while others do not. Our reaction depends in part on how full our rainbarrel is at the time of the stress.[62]

CHAPTER 8

Necessary Nutrients

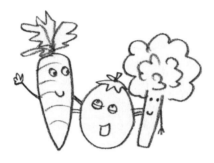

The subject of minerals and vitamins is highly complex. The published literature and documentation covering these essential substances is voluminous and frequently contentious. For these reasons, this book is not the place for an extended examination of minerals and vitamins. There are, however, a small handful that are worthy of familiarisation, as the effects of deficiencies of these substances are often acutely felt by people with PBS.

Fats

Many people regard fat as a bad thing. However, the truth is more complex than that as fats come in many forms. While some of these are, indeed, undeniably bad, others are essential for our health – as is striking the right balance between them.

Essential fatty acids, most notably omega 3 and omega 6, support cellular metabolic function. As our bodies don't produce these fats, it's vital that they form part of our diet, hence the term 'essential' fatty acids.

The essential fatty acids balancing act

In an ideal diet, the ratio of omega 6 to omega 3 is 1:1. In reality, most people on diets that are high in processed or fast foods are way off this target. High in omega 6, yet low in omega 3, the oils these foods are cooked in are likely to give these people an actual ratio of up to 20:1. Another factor in this imbalance is the reduced omega 3 content in milk which is produced from cows that are fed on corn or soya.

Good sources of omega 3 are:

- algae (some are high in omega 3)
- dark leafy vegetables
- eggs (free range and not fed on soya)
- flaxseed
- walnuts.

I also recognise that fish and fish oils are rich in omega 3 but I advise you be careful of the sources that you use. They are also invariably high in mercury, something that is bad for anyone and especially so for people managing PBS.

Extra virgin olive oil provides moderate quantities of both omega 6 and omega 3, but only if consumed uncooked. A consequence of heating any cooking oil, no matter how pure or how expensive, is the creation of toxins. This is why almost every health practitioner advises against diets high in fried food. Where frying is unavoidable, opt for coconut oil or ghee.

Saturated fats – the fats of life

Natural saturated fats, such as butter, meat fats, coconut oil and palm oil are the subject of opposing beliefs. In conventional medicine they are considered to be a factor in heart disease, cancer, obesity, diabetes, malfunction of cell membranes and multiple sclerosis. However, there is a lot of evidence to support the theory that the real damage is done by processed liquid vegetable oils and artificially hardened vegetable oils, known as trans fats.

We need saturated fats and we need them in the stiffness that their natural, solid form provides. In liquid form, they make the cell membranes floppy, while in the artificial trans fat form, they stiffen the membranes. Both these states compromise the membranes' structural integrity and capacity to function.

Our lungs, nervous system and heart depend on saturated fats and even half of the fat in the brain is saturated. Natural saturated fats are also known to:

- support kidney function
- aid hormone production
- strengthen the immune system
- protect against cancer
- protect against diabetes by supporting the insulin receptors
- suppress inflammation
- carry the vital vitamins A, D and K2.

Hydrogenated oils

Many processed and packaged foods are cooked using oils that are hydrogenated or partially hydrogenated. Hydrogenation makes these oils last longer and withstand higher cooking temperatures.

As I mentioned above, heating oil to high temperatures is harmful enough. However, hydrogenation ruins any nutritious value the oil may have had in the first place by creating trans fatty acids. These reduce the absorption of nutrients and allow toxins to build up in our cells.

Always check the labels of foods for fats, and remember: natural saturated fats and a diet that gives you a 1:1 ratio of omega 6 to omega 3 (or as close as you can get) are good; artificial fats, trans fats and hydrogenated fats are bad.

Magnesium

Magnesium deficiency is extremely common, particularly in those with PBS. Modern farming techniques have seen to it that magnesium levels in soil are depleted and this is compounded by the increase in the consumption of refined and processed foods. Put bluntly, most of us struggle to reach the EU recommended daily allowance (RDA) of magnesium in our diet: 375mg, and 450mg for pregnant and breastfeeding mothers. When you consider that just 100 years ago the average diet contained four times today's RDA, the degeneration in quality of the most commonly consumed foods, in nutritious terms at least, is stark.

Magnesium has many functions. Of most interest to people with PBS, however, are that it helps to relax muscles, activates B vitamins, supports hormone production and promotes detoxification, in particular helping to flush heavy metals from the cells. Magnesium is also necessary for sufficient energy levels.

Conversely, then, a magnesium deficiency can result in several symptoms, including chronic fatigue, migraines, depression and muscle cramps and tremors. Over time, severe lack of magnesium can trigger a dangerous chain of events starting with permeability in the walls of the body's cells. This leads to the loss of potassium and other minerals, allowing sodium and calcium to take their place. If the build-up of calcium becomes excessive, it can cause kidney stones. As we have seen, if kidney health is compromised, impurities that are otherwise filtered out may remain in the urine, where, upon reaching the bladder, they can cause the classic PBS symptoms of pain, frequency and urgency. (The ideal ratio of calcium and magnesium in the body is 2:1.) In tests on rats, magnesium deficiency has been shown to compromise the autoimmune system.

Many tests for magnesium deficiency are conducted by analysing a sample of your urine, sweat or blood. I find this too simplistic, however; rather than the serum test, which measures how much magnesium is floating in the blood stream, the red cell test actually tells us how much magnesium is in the cells (see 'Testing for magnesium deficiency' in Chapter 9).

Magnesium needs to be kept at regulated levels and in balance with calcium. For some people with deficiencies and other biochemical factors, this can mean taking more than the RDA in order to redress an imbalance. Magnesium can be taken safely in a range of forms. Foods that contain magnesium include:

- chlorella

- eggs

- fish

- green vegetables

- nuts (especially almonds)

- pulses

- pumkin seeds

- seaweeds

- spirulina

- wheatgrass.

If you have an intolerance to any of the foods above or have been advised to avoid any for PBS-related reasons you may find your options narrowed down somewhat. You can take a magnesium citrate supplement, although if that irritates your bladder then magnesium oil can be rubbed into the skin, or you can try a magnesium bath once a week, to begin to replenish your levels.

Health food shops, supermarkets and online supplement stores provide a range of magnesium supplements in powder and capsule form while homeopathic remedies such as Mag Phos help the body absorb the mineral from foods. The same is true with black pepper with meals as this helps with the absorption of anything it is eaten with.

Do not take magnesium supplements if you have any form of kidney disease.

If your condition or dietary regime prevent you from boosting your magnesium levels orally, you can still remedy a deficiency by taking a good long soak in an Epsom salts bath. Lying in a warm bath containing 1 per cent Epsom salts (magnesium sulphate), which is around 500–600 grams for a typical domestic tub, allows you to absorb magnesium through the skin easily and safely. In recent years more and more research has been conducted into magnesium baths. No dangerous side-effects have been identified.

Diana, age 64

Diana, a long-term PBS patient, had been experiencing migraines sporadically for 30 years.

For Diana a migraine could strike at any time, but after keeping a diary she noticed that they coincided with periods of emotional stress and PBS flare-ups. 'I began to realise that migraines were part of a vicious circle,' she says. 'The pain and discomfort in my bladder and pelvic area generally would get me on an emotional low at times and it appeared that this triggered the migraine.'

Conventional medicine and strong prescription painkillers failed to kill the pain, so Diana turned her attention to the underlying causes.

A red cell test revealed a magnesium deficiency. Immediately, Diana started taking magnesium in the form of Epsom salts baths. Within months she discovered that her migraines had ceased, even during her PBS flare-ups. Three years on this remains the case.

Vitamin B12

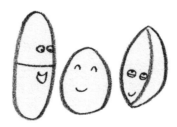

Vitamin B12 is essential to a range of bodily functions such as DNA replication and the metabolism of amino acids and fats. It's also vital to detoxification and, therefore, a vital nutrient in the diet of anyone with PBS. And yet, like magnesium, vitamin B12 deficiencies are common in these types of patient.

There are two main reasons for vitamin B12 deficiency. First, it is present exclusively in animal products, making it absent from the diets of vegans and vegetarians. Second, there are a number of conditions that impair the body's ability to absorb vitamin B12. The list includes bacterial infections in the gut and mercury in the gut. As these are common in people with PBS, it follows that your practitioner will probably recommend that you are tested for vitamin B12 deficiency (see Chapter 9), especially if you have any of the classic psychological or neurological symptoms, which include (but are not limited to):

- apathy

- confusion

- depression

- memory loss

- mood swings

- pain

- tremors.

Other ways in which vitamin B12 deficiency can make itself felt are through chronic fatigue, disturbed appetite, constipation and diarrhoea, insomnia, repeated infections and tongue soreness.

Of course, all these symptoms can be caused by many other conditions so another good reason for the vitamin B12 deficiency test is to rule these factors out.

Once tested, your practitioner will be able to advise you how to increase your intake of vitamin B12 if necessary. While the RDA is 1.5mcg per day, the reduced absorption that affects many people with PBS means that I frequently recommend a higher intake in order to compensate. This can range from 50mcg right up to 2000mcg per day, depending on test results.

After animal products, the most commonly used sources of vitamin B12 are dietary supplements sold in health food shops, supermarkets and online stores. Other options include a skin patch or, for extreme cases, high dose injections. Always consult a qualified practitioner before taking any supplement whose dosage exceeds the RDA.

Janet, age 43

Janet, a vegetarian of 20 years, arrived at my clinic complaining of fatigue, depression, menstrual irregularity, poor memory and phases of hair loss. She had also recently been craving meat. Tests by Janet's doctor had shown her full blood count to be normal with no anaemia detected. She was referred to a psychiatrist. When I met Janet, it was clear that she had several health issues, including a fungal dysbiosis in her gut and nerve pain in her bladder. I suspected she was low in vitamin B12 so recommended a test. The result was within the normal limits, albeit at the bottom end of the scale at 206pg/ml. As well as adjusting Janet's diet, I recommended that she start a programme of high dosage B12 supplements in liquid form taken sublingually (under the tongue) every day and a retest after three months.

The second test showed an increase in Janet's B12 level to 350pg/ml. She reported a dramatic increase in energy, cessation of hair loss and bladder pain and a great improvement in her mental wellbeing. However, due to the possible long-term depletion in her B12 levels, Janet agreed to continue with the high dosage B12 supplement for a further 18 months to replenish her levels.

B12 is a common deficiency which is easily missed. I believe that the bladder discomfort was neurological because of the B12 deficiency, and fortunately she was able to take the supplement without aggravating her urinary symptoms, which isn't always the case.

Zinc

Zinc is another mineral with particular significance to PBS patients. Zinc is necessary for the production of stomach acid, the correct quantity and pH of which ensure that foods are broken down properly so as not to damage the bladder wall. It is also vital to the immune system and, in conjunction with vitamins A, B6, C and E, helps to alleviate allergic reactions.

Unfortunately, almost every patient I see has a shortage of zinc. This can lead to a variety of emotional as well as physical symptoms and disorders including:

- depression

- anxiety

- psychiatric disorders

- hormonal imbalances

- immune problems

- insufficient hydrochloric acid levels

- digestive disturbances.

Testing for deficiency is tricky as zinc resides within the cells of the body. However, skin problems such as dryness or flakiness are possible early indications of a shortage as the body will take zinc stored from the skin when vital levels are low. Other signs that there's not enough zinc in the body are general fatigue and increased susceptibility to infection.

Good sources of zinc are alfalfa sprouts, nettles and seeds, especially pumpkin and sunflower seeds. You'll also find zinc supplements at the supermarket, health food shops and online stores in capsule and, at some retailers, liquid form. Bear in mind that zinc can affect the body's ability to absorb copper. So, if you do opt to take a zinc supplement or your practitioner recommends it, seek advice on taking a copper supplement too.

The EU RDA for zinc is 10mg; higher for pregnant and breastfeeding women. If someone is low in zinc then usually a supplement providing 30mg daily is enough to deal with a deficiency. Always consult a qualified practitioner before taking any supplement whose dosage exceeds the RDA.

Antioxidants

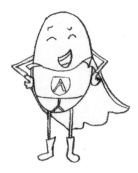

Antioxidants help to maintain the balance of the immune system by scavenging free radicals. They can attack free radicals in several ways from preventing them from forming in the first place to interrupting their processes and reducing the energy they contain.

Many effective antioxidants are produced in the body itself. These are superoxide dismutase, catalase and glutathione peroxidase. Additional sources of antioxidants are many and varied and include:

- *vitamin, mineral and enzyme-rich foods,* especially those high in vitamin C, vitamin E, beta-carotene, lutein, lycopene, vitamin B2, co-enzyme Q10 and the amino acid cysteine

- *herbs,* including bilberry, turmeric, grape seed and pine bark extracts

- *superfoods,* such as mangosteen, kombucha, açaí, pomegranate, goji berry, chia seed and spirulina

- *supplements:* for the best results, choose manganese, zinc, copper and selenium. However these shouldn't be taken ad hoc but according to what your practitioner discovers through appropriate testing. They support the body's own antioxidant production process and are more easily absorbed than ready-made antioxidant products.

Many antioxidants, particularly when used in combinations, also have powerful anti-inflammatory properties. If you experience chronic or painful inflammatory disorders (i.e. anything ending in 'itis', such as cystitis) ask your practitioner for advice on the best combination for you.

FREE RADICALS

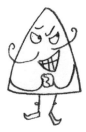

Free radicals are cells that contain 'extra' energy, which can only be used up if they attack other cells in the body. When this attack takes place, the assaulted cell is compromised. Over a period of time, free radicals can be a contributory factor in the development of cancer and accelerate the ageing process.

Free radicals can be produced by the body through its regular metabolism or ingested by exposure to pollution and other harmful chemicals in our environment. These include ionising radiation from x-rays, industrial processes and the sun; cosmic rays; heavy metals such as mercury, cadmium and lead; cigarette smoke; alcohol; and rancid oils.

CHAPTER 9

Testing

In order to determine whether you are indeed being affected by toxicity such as mercury, or have leaky gut or adrenal fatigue, then the practitioner you are working with may want to undertake certain diagnostics.

Testing for mercury

The presence of excess mercury in the body can be detected by analysing two urine samples produced either side of taking the chelating agent dimercaptosuccinic acid (DMSA (Kelmer)).

A chelating agent is a substance that binds to a target in the body, in this case mercury. Mercury is known to be difficult to excrete. This is one of the reasons it is so dangerous, and also why meaningful levels of the metal rarely show up in standard urine tests. DSMA (Kelmer) binds the mercury and is passed in the urine. So, by comparing the before-and-after urine samples, it's possible to discover if there are hidden mercury levels in the body beyond those attributed to normal background exposure.

Your part in the mercury test

- Collect urine sample No. 1 early in the morning – around 8.00am.

- Immediately after collecting urine sample No. 1, take the DSMA (Kelmer) capsules. The dosage of the capsules will have been measured specifically for you based on your body weight – around 15mg per kg.

- After 2½ hours collect urine sample No. 2. Ignore any urine passed in the meantime.

- Label your urine sample containers clearly before returning for analysis.

If the level of mercury in urine sample No. 2 is double that of No. 1 your practitioner will advise you that mercury levels are excessive and recommend ways to reduce your exposure to the metal and detoxify.

Though DSMA is safe (unless you are pregnant or breastfeeding), if you have – or think you have – white cell sensitivity to metals, this form of testing may not be recommended. Similarly, some patients with PBS may experience a reaction due to the additional mercury entering the bladder in the urine. In this case, a urine test without taking the capsules will avert the symptoms, although the results won't be quite so accurate.

Test results typically take around five days to arrive.

Testing for adrenal hormone levels

Through the production of the hormones cortisol and dehydroepiandrosterone, the adrenal glands are responsible for controlling our response to mental and emotional stress, anxiety and fear. And though cortisol levels fluctuate throughout the day, levels of both hormones are present in our saliva. This means that assessing our capacity for dealing with stress can be tested by analysing saliva samples taken at four points throughout the day that reflect the changing levels of cortisol during our waking hours. The adrenal hormone saliva test can also help to uncover causes of conditions such as chronic fatigue, depression and insomnia and diseases including diabetes.

Your part in the adrenal hormone saliva test
All you need to do is spit into a container four times in a single day. The times are:

- early morning – around 8.00am

- mid-day – around 12.00 noon

- afternoon – around 4.00pm

- night – between 11.00pm and 12.00 midnight.

There's no need to refrigerate your samples so the test should fit easily into your schedule. Once you have your samples ready, label the containers as described on your kit and return for analysis. The results take around two weeks to come back, so arrange a convenient appointment with your practitioner who will help you interpret your findings.

Although many doctors are unconvinced about – or unaware of – the accuracy and reliability of adrenal hormone saliva tests, they are recognised by the World Health Organisation (WHO). I have found them to be highly valuable in working with patients who have conditions that are exacerbated by stress and anxiety, of which PBS is a prime example.

Testing for a leaky gut

Detecting permeability in the gut is possible by way of a process known as the polyethylene glycol (PEG) test. Polyethylene glycol (PEG 400) is a substance that the body has no use for and, therefore, will not absorb for the purpose of any bodily function. This means that, when consumed as a drink made up of known molecular composition, a healthy gut will allow some of the small molecules through its wall and into the urine, while blocking the larger molecules, which end up in the faeces. A leaky gut, on the other hand, will allow the large and the small molecules to pass through. By analysing urine produced after drinking PEG, doctors can determine the size of the molecules in the sample and, by extension, the permeability of the gut wall.

Your part in the PEG

- First, empty your bladder.

- Drink the peg 400 solution.

- Collect all the urine you produce over the next six hours.

At the laboratory, analysts will be able to identify the size of the PEG 400 molecules in your urine sample. The presence of the larger molecules indicates that the gut has increased permeability. Results are typically ready in seven days.

Testing for yeast overgrowth

Another test, the gut fermentation study, can detect if you have an overgrowth of yeast in your gut. Quite simply, you take a sugary capsule or drink and provide a blood sample one hour later. If there is excessive yeast in the gut, it will ferment the sugar in the capsule/drink and convert it to alcohol. The alcohol will then show up in the blood test.

The gut fermentation study can also identify low dietary fibre and possible hypoglycaemia and give practitioners an overview of the balance of the flora in the bowel.

A stool test is another way that a yeast overgrowth can be detected. This can also be helpful in determining the exact strain of yeast or bacteria present as well as the type and strain of beneficial bacteria potentially absent.

Testing for magnesium deficiency

The red cell magnesium test measures the amount of magnesium in your red blood cells. This is a far more accurate gauge of your real magnesium levels than a serum test as heart function depends on keeping the serum magnesium at levels within tight upper and lower parameters. So, as long as your heart is beating, it stands to reason that a serum test will show normal levels. However, as the serum levels are adjusted by extracting magnesium from the red blood cells, this test gives us the real picture.

Your part in the red cell magnesium test
The red cell test is carried out by analysing your blood. You will need a make an appointment with a phlebotomist who will extract the required sample and send it to the analysing laboratory. When the test result is returned, arrange to see your practitioner who will explain the results and give you advice on how to correct any deficiency.

Testing for vitamin B12 deficiency

A B12 serum blood test is the standard way to determine the levels of B12 someone has in their blood. It is useful as a general guide and will reveal if someone has pernicious anaemia. However, the most effective means of detecting a vitamin B12 deficiency is the MMA (methylmalonic acid) test.

MMA is a waste product that builds up in the blood. Where a person has adequate levels of vitamin B12, MMA is converted into a substance called succinic acid. Where there is a deficiency of vitamin B12 MMA is passed into the urine. MMA can be present within ten days of the onset of the deficiency.

Your part in the MMA test

You can have either your blood or your urine sample tested for MMA, depending upon which service your health care provider offers. Both are very reliable and the levels of any MMA detected will reflect the extent of the deficiency they indicate.

Testing for toxins

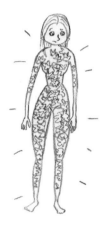

The most dangerous toxins that people can have are the external toxins in our environment that get inside a person's body and to their DNA. Known as DNA adducts, these can affect the structure and shape of DNA and compromise their capacity to replicate, repair and express themselves. This, in turn, can severely affect a range of body functions. DNA adducts are commonplace in people with cancer and neurological diseases such as Parkinson's disease. People who are told that their symptoms are simply unexplainable and are given a diagnosis of chronic fatigue also usually test positive for DNA adducts.

Common examples of DNA adducts in people with PBS that I treat are hair dye, heavy metals, plastics and volatile organic compounds (VOCs) such as formaldehyde.

This test enables doctors and practitioners to detect and measure a wide range of substances that can become DNA adducts and the genes they adhere to. It is a blood test which involves sending a few millilitres to a laboratory.

Urine broth culture

The urine broth culture is a liquid medium for studying the growth of bacteria in urine over an extended period of time. A much slower method of cultivating bacteria than the standard urine analysis, this method provides a more accurate replica of the internal bladder conditions than the standard urinary tract infection (UTI) test. With the temperature closely controlled and monitored, the broth culture enables the urine to evolve as it would do in the body over a longer period. This can reveal the presence of infections that would remain hidden in the shorter analysis and therefore remain untreated.

The subject of the urine broth culture is not without controversy. Many practitioners in orthodox medicine maintain that the conventional rapid culture test will show all bacteria in the urine. Many patients, however, are left bewildered by repeated negative results when their symptoms suggest otherwise. I have personally carried out the urine broth culture on occasions and believe in its value.

Ways to detoxify
Skin brushing

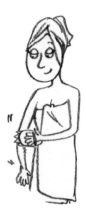

Skin brushing boosts the immune system and enhances organ function through improved circulation and flow of qi (energy) through the body's energy network channels. It will also have an excellent effect on your complexion and muscle tone and help you feel revitalised.

Skin brushing kick-starts the metabolism so it will work best as part of your morning routine.

BEFORE YOU GET STARTED
Buy a skin brush from your local body care shop. Avoid synthetic bristles as these will produce static electricity, which is both unpleasant and unhealthy. I find that cactus fibres make the best bristles. Although they are quite firm when new, they will soften with use.

HOW TO SKIN BRUSH
Your skin needs to be dry for optimum detoxification so allow between five and ten minutes before showering, bathing or washing.

Don't brush delicate or irritated skin, varicose veins or any areas affected by eczema of psoriasis.

Always brush towards your heart.

Start at the soles of your feet to activate the reflexology points, then brush from your toes towards your ankles over your upper foot.

Now brush your legs vigorously, paying particular attention to lymphatic glands around your ankles, the back of the knees and your groin. Give them all at least five or six thorough strokes.

Continue upwards over your thighs and buttocks but avoid the genital area. When you reach your abdomen, use circular clockwise brush strokes. To begin with, make three to four circular movements, then gradually increase this to 12 over the next few days.

Next, brush the insides and outsides of your hands and then the same for both arms. Keep the strokes long and always in the direction of your heart. Pay special attention to the inside of the elbows and the armpits.

A decent skin brush will be too uncomfortable to use on your face, but don't forget the sides and back of neck. Also include your chest but avoid the nipples. Brush as much of your upper back and shoulders as you can reach.

To get the maximum benefit from your skin brush, follow it up with a hot and cold shower.

For the first two to three months, skin brush daily, then reduce the frequency to every other day. This will keep the therapy effective without your body getting too used to it.

Wash your brush regularly with warm water and essential oils such as tea tree to keep it clean and free of bacteria. Then, be sure to dry it thoroughly to prevent mould growth and ensure no one else uses it.

Far infrared saunas (FIRS)

Far infrared rays are an important component of the sun's rays. They warm our skin when we sit in direct sunlight and penetrate through the skin and mobilise subcutaneous tissues. These are then excreted through sweat. All this happens without our body heat rising, which means that we can eliminate unwanted chemicals more safely. It also means that patients unable to use conventional saunas for health reasons are more likely to be able to tolerate, and therefore benefit from, a far infrared sauna.

Anyone with a medical condition, such as heart disease, should consult a qualified practitioner before using any type of sauna.

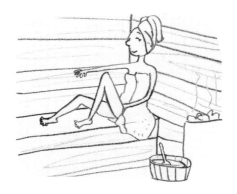

USING A FAR INFRARED SAUNA

The best results from far infrared saunas come from several short sessions on a regular basis rather than long sessions with long intervals between. A good programme to start with would be to take two sessions a week and build up to a session every day.

Once the skin has started to sweat, you will have had the full benefit of the far infrared sauna. The toxic chemicals will now be on the surface of your skin and will need to be showered off to prevent them from being reabsorbed back into the body. By the next day, chemicals in the deeper tissues will be passing into the superficial layers and you'll be ready to repeat the far infrared process and detoxify further. After a few weeks of the programme, toxic chemicals will gradually be drawn out from even deeper layers and expelled from your body through your skin.

Remember, when you sweat you excrete good as well as bad chemicals. This means it's important to rehydrate and to replace the lost minerals. There are a number of mineral replacement products on the market – ask your practitioner to recommend the best one for you.

Taking before-and-after fat biopsies or blood tests will enable your practitioner to monitor your progress during far infrared saunas. In this way, it's possible to detoxify effectively without overburdening the liver and kidneys.

There is a wide range of far infrared saunas available on the market, from small portable devices that you can use in your home to custom-made installations. Prices start at less than £200. If you have internet access, simply search 'far infrared saunas' to see all the options. Alternatively, ask your practitioner for advice.

Castor oil packs

Castor oil packs are excellent for people with PBS as they are soothing, anti-inflammatory and help to provide relief to the muscles around the pelvic floor. They are also a highly effective form of detoxification as they draw toxins out of the body through the skin. Many people with PBS use castor oil packs as part of their strategy for reducing the intensity of flare-ups.

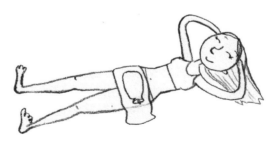

When taken internally, castor oil is a highly effective treatment for constipation. For detoxifying, however, it's applied externally on the skin, so there are no bowel movement related side-effects! As well as PBS, detoxifying through castor oil packs can help the immune system, viral conditions, glandular fever, gynaecological problems, bowel disorders, scars and adhesions and problems associated with the nervous system.

MAKING AND USING A CASTOR OIL PACK
You will need:

- 5–6 tablespoons good quality, cold pressed castor oil
- soft flannel made of cotton or wool (not dyed or bleached)
- hot water bottle
- small saucepan.

Gently heat the castor oil in a non-aluminium pan to a temperature which is not too hot to touch. Soak the flannel in the castor oil and place over your pelvis. Cover the flannel with a towel and place a hot water bottle on top. Now, simply lie down for 45 minutes to an hour. Listening to music or simply enjoying the silence can enhance relaxation. Focus your mind on the drawing out of toxins that is now happening.

You can wash the oil off later or even the next morning if you fall asleep, or you may prefer to clean it off straight away. To ensure that the toxins are not reabsorbed back into your body, wash the area where the pack has been with a mixture of 2½ teaspoons of baking soda and a litre of warm water. Clean a second time with ordinary soap if necessary.

You (and only you) can use the flannel for up to 30 applications. It is not usually possible to wash all of the oil from the flannel, so make sure you store the flannel in a container in the fridge between sessions to keep any residual oil in the fabric fresh. To use the flannel again, warm up the oil in a pan and soak the flannel as before.

You can make your castor oil pack as warm as you wish. A temperature that provides relief to one person may be unbearably hot for another. There's no prescribed temperature, so experiment to find the heat level that works for you.

CHAPTER 10

Taking the Fear Out of Flare-ups

Most people with PBS will have flare-ups at some stage, though the intensity, frequency and duration of the experience can vary enormously from person to person. They are the result of the bladder wall becoming more inflamed than usual or the pelvic floor muscles going into spasm. Typically, though not always, a flare-up is a response to known triggers such as foods, sex, hormonal changes, cycling or sitting down during long journeys (see below).

As I mentioned in the introduction, the PBS symptoms of pain, frequency and urgency temporarily intensify during a flare-up. As well as (and because of) the physical discomfort this causes, flare-ups can seriously affect a patient's quality of life through lost sleep and restricted capacity to work, socialise or enjoy intimacy.

As well as a great deal of distress, flare-ups can also cause confusion by masquerading as urinary tract infections (UTIs). They share the symptoms of frequency, urgency, pain and night-time discomfort. It's not uncommon for GPs to mistakenly put patients on antibiotics each time a flare-up occurs when, in fact, no infection is present. In a study of 106 PBS patients by Edward Stanford and colleagues looking into this issue,[63] only one patient in 15 (less than 7%) had recurring UTIs – the rest were experiencing regular PBS flare-ups.

That said, if you suspect you have a bladder infection I strongly urge you to have a urine test. Similarly, always see your GP if you have blood in your urine or experience back pain or a fever, and never leave symptoms beyond those you normally experience during a flare-up unchecked.

Most commonly, the fuller a PBS patient's bladder becomes during a flare-up, the worse the pain is. Urinating, while also painful, soothes this for a short period, but often not for long and nor does it always relieve the sensation of a full bladder. This is because an inflamed bladder feels similar to a full one. Where PBS has affected a person's pelvic floor muscles, the pain is more of a constant ache due to the muscles going into spasm. Relaxing the muscles to allow for urination can be difficult, while a build-up of lactic acid can also contribute to the pain and general sensation of tightness and heaviness in the region. Less commonly, people can also experience fasciculation during a flare. This is a vibrating sensation caused by pressure on the pudendal nerve, one of the main nerves in the pelvic region affecting the bladder, sphincter, rectum and genitalia of both sexes. Pain felt during flare-ups can also spread to the thighs and lower back area.

How long a flare-up lasts varies enormously from person to person. For some patients, it may be a few hours, for others, weeks or months. It's impossible to predict as the nature of PBS varies greatly across patients, as does each individual's sensitivity to triggers. It may be reasonable to presume, however, that there is a correlation between the severity of a given patient's PBS and the length and intensity of his or her flare-ups.

PBS flare-up triggers

Acidic foods and drinks, those containing histamines, artificial sugars and vitamin supplements:

- coffee (caffeinated or decaffeinated)
- tea (regular and green, hot or iced)
- alcohol (especially wine)
- carbonated drinks
- fruit juices: especially orange juice, cranberry juice, lemon juice and tomato juice
- chocolate: especially the cheap brands of milk chocolate
- aspartame: an artificial sweetener used in products such as NutraSweet.

Medications:

- multivitamins: especially vitamin C and vitamin B6
- ibuprofen
- antibiotics
- steroids
- the contraceptive pill.

Hormonal changes, especially during menstruation and ovulation:

- increased progesterone levels in some patients
- increased oestrogen levels in others.

Stress: physical and emotional:

- exposure to cold
- constipation

- car journeys, due to extended jarring from bumpy roads and long periods in a sitting position
- train journeys and flights, due to limited or difficult access to lavatories
- exercise, such as cycling, swimming and other activities that strain or apply pressure to the pelvic area
- mental and emotional stress
- sex, through friction and increased muscle activity.

Exposure to toxins:

- vehicle fumes
- soaps, bubble baths, detergents
- chlorine in swimming pools
- smoking: the by-products of cigarette smoke are processed by the kidney and pass through the bladder before being excreted
- Volatile organic compounds (VOCs), such as from paint, new carpets.

Creating a flare-up control strategy

In this section I have outlined the most commonly used methods for both preventing PBS flare-ups and minimising their effects when they occur. Not all of them will necessarily work for you and some may be far more effective than others. However, by experimenting and combining those that work best for you, you can formulate your personal PBS flare-up defence strategy. Whatever strategy you devise, be ready to act early – nipping a flare-up in the bud is the key to making the plan effective.

Relax

If possible, sit or lie down to allow the pelvic muscles to relax. They may have gone into spasm. Heat pads placed over the bladder and pelvis can help the muscles to relax, as can taking a warm bath. Avoid adding bubble bath, salts or anything scented to the bath water as the chemicals they contain often cause irritation. Instead use baking powder for a soothing effect.

Dilute the urine and reduce acid levels

Watered down urine is far less irritating to the bladder wall than urine with high concentrations of toxins. Drink plenty of water and keep an eye on the colour of your urine. If it's clear to pale yellow, that's fine. If it's dark yellow or cloudy, keep drinking. Adding ½ teaspoon of baking powder to a glass of water will reduce the acid level in your urine and alleviate bladder pain. This is not recommended if you are on a salt-reduced diet or have high blood pressure. A safe alternative to baking powder is the commercially available Prelief (see page 88).

Calm and soothe the bladder wall

As well as avoiding the trigger foods and drinks listed above, ensure that your diet includes foods that soothe the bladder wall. These include chicken, potatoes, rice, carrots, mushrooms and squashes. Peppermint tea and camomile tea have antispasmodic qualities and will also help with pelvic muscle pain.

Supplementing your diet with a personalised herbal regime can also help to soothe the bladder wall and reduce the intensity of flare-ups. A qualified herbalist will be able to assess your circumstances and prescribe the right blend of herbs and dosage specifically for you.

Relax the pelvic muscles
There is a wide range of exercises that you can do to relax muscles in the pelvic floor and relieve tension. These include deep breathing, stretching and applying pressure to specific trigger points to release tension. A professional therapist will be able to prepare an exercise plan that is convenient and safe for you to carry out at home.

Minimise your intake of bladder irritants
If you can, avoid taking antibiotics, steroids and pain relievers such as ibuprofen. If you use the contraceptive pill, spermicides or a diaphragm, you may find changing to a non-chemical contraceptive helps your flare-ups. And if you smoke, try to cut down or, even better, quit altogether as this will drastically reduce the toxins passing into your bladder.

Plan your travelling
If your lifestyle involves a lot of travelling, devise journey plans that allow time for plenty of toilet stops. On trains and aircraft, take steps to ensure you are seated near to the toilets. If you drive extensively, buy the most comfortable car you can afford. Taking a muscle relaxant before setting off may alleviate the effects of driving over bumps and sitting in the same position for long periods.

Manage stress
Of course, this is easier said than done as most causes of stress are beyond our power to control. However, through complex mechanisms in the brain and spinal cord, mental and emotional stress converts into pain in the pelvic region. If possible, seek help in developing ways to reduce or manage stress and anxiety.

Sit with a castor oil pack

Castor oil packs soothe and relieve pain in the pelvic muscles. Sitting for 45 minutes to an hour with a flannel soaked in heated castor oil and covered with a hot water bottle can help enormously as part of your flare-up control strategy. And, while you enjoy the calming effect of a castor oil pack session, you'll also be detoxifying your pelvic area too. See pages 142–144 for full instructions on preparing and using a castor oil pack.

Dealing with thrush, vaginal and urethra irritation

If someone is suffering from repeated urinary tract infections as well as thrush, this can be a helpful procedure.

Insert two probiotic capsules vaginally overnight. In an hour they will usually dissolve, flooding the area with beneficial bacteria. This is particularly useful with an outbreak of thrush and irritation affecting the vagina and entry to the bladder. This can be repeated for as long as necessary. Be mindful to avoid intercourse within 12 hours of inserting a probiotic capsule.

Gill, age 26

Shortly after qualifying as a teacher, Gill began to develop urinary incontinence. As well as emotionally upsetting, the physical discomfort made teaching particularly difficult. So stressed was Gill that she considered quitting her job.

With no infection detected in any tests, Gill's doctor believed her problem was related to her pelvic floor muscles. When exercising these muscles had no effect, she was diagnosed with overactive bladder. Again, suggested treatments failed to improve Gill's symptoms.

After 18 months during which her symptoms worsened and her stress levels increased, Gill, who enjoys a glass of wine, read an article about how diet, and in particular alcohol and coffee, can aggravate bladder problems. She cut out both and noticed a difference in days.

Gill continues to do pelvic floor exercises and pilates, which she believes helps her symptoms. But she's in no doubt that cutting out wine and coffee made the biggest difference.

Trauma release exercises

Trauma and mental and emotional stress can manifest itself into a physiological issue. Physical cells in the muscles across the body – and in particular the pelvic region – hold memory of unresolved trauma in the form of toxins which get released at times of anxiety. These toxins then contribute to the assault on the bladder and the pain experienced by people with PBS. The problem is compounded by the fact that, when our bodies experience anxiety, they instinctively seek to protect themselves from further distress. In so doing, they erect a barrier to healing processes. This condition is commonplace in PBS patients that I treat so, unsurprisingly, breaking down these barriers by releasing chronic tension and stagnation in the pelvic area is essential to a person's recovery plan.

To help us expel this trauma, there are exercises that, in effect, put the body into trauma and trigger our on-board trauma release mechanism, shaking. To achieve the ultimate aim of releasing the harmful toxins associated with stored stress, the exercises force us to engage well-established traumatic patterns in the body. These type of exercises were originally advocated by the influential Austrian psychiatrist and psychoanalyst, Wilhelm Reich (1897–1957). The most recent proponent is the highly respected American traumatologist and author, David Berceli PhD, who incorporated the exercises into his 2008 book, *The Revolutionary Trauma Release Process.*[64]

The Trauma Release Process™ triggers the body's shaking mechanism. This stimulates contractions in the seven thigh flexor muscles, also known as hip flexors. The main exercise that I use with my patients engages the body's natural tremor mechanisms, starting a process of shaking from the body's centre of gravity, the pelvis. From here, the shaking begins to reverberate and spread across the whole of the body, travelling through the thighs, the psoas muscle and lower back, then up the spine and into the shoulders, neck, arms and hands. As it moves through the body, the shaking flushes out stored tension in the muscles and returns them to a relaxed state.

As well as helping to expel long-term trauma, regular shaking can prevent the more minor anxieties and commonplace emotional challenges of today from escalating into the stored stress of tomorrow. Because the way the body shakes in the exercises prescribed in the Trauma Release Process™ is completely natural, there's no reason why you cannot build them into an existing fitness regime or practise them at home.

Responses to shaking vary. For some people they are energising, for others exhausting. Similarly, the duration of the exercise you can tolerate and the intensity of the response to the exercises is different for each individual. This is because shaking can evoke powerful emotional responses, particularly in people harbouring long-term stress and unresolved trauma. This is quite normal – it is, after all, the objective of the shaking exercise to release these emotions and free you of them once and for all. However, rather than allow yourself to be overwhelmed, simply slow down and do the exercises at the rate that you find manageable. Once you have found your pace and settled into your optimum shaking regime, you will feel more emotionally stable as well as physically more supple.

On the other hand, don't feel cheated or think that you're doing it incorrectly if you don't respond emotionally to shaking. We're all unique, with different emotional make-ups, histories and tension patterns. Accordingly, there is no one correct way of shaking or reacting to shaking – your body will determine for itself exactly how it needs to shake. If you shake vigorously at first, this would suggest that your tremors have encountered large amounts of tension. Once these have been broken down, the intensity of your shaking will settle down and make way for more gentle vibrations. Fluctuations in the way you shake are nothing to panic about, nor are varying patterns of shaking that may emerge. Trust your body, listen to its signals and very soon you will instinctively know when and how to purge stress.

To begin with, these exercises are usually carried out on alternate days for the first month. This will give your body a good introduction to shaking as a form of trauma release and begin to loosen the muscles. In the second month, you can reduce the frequency to two days a week, though this is the minimum I would recommend to prevent stress building back up again. Over time you will find that the benefits of shaking exercises accumulate as they reach deeper and deeper into the muscles.

If you find the emotional release from shaking too difficult to withstand, or experience any physical discomfort, stop immediately and seek professional help. A qualified practitioner will offer supervision and help you tailor your exercise regime to your personal circumstances.

David Berceli sets out six shaking exercises in the Trauma Release Process™. This is the one I find most helpful for releasing trauma related to PBS (if you are uncomfortable at any time, stop the exercise by straightening your legs and relaxing on the floor):

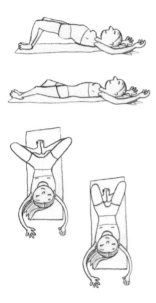

- *Step 1*: Lie with your feet together and your knees relaxing in as open a position as possible.

- *Step 2*: Raise your pelvis by two inches for one minute, keeping your knees open and relaxed. Don't worry about your arms – position them where they are most comfortable for you.

- *Step 3*: Rest your pelvis back down on the floor and relax for one minute. You may now feel your legs starting to shake.

- *Step 4*: Adjust your knees so they are two inches above their relaxed open position. Lie in this position for two minutes. The quivering may become stronger. If it's comfortable, let it continue.

- *Step 5*: Bring your knees another two inches closer together and feel the shaking spread to your legs. The quivering will become stronger. Bring your knees two inches closer still and allow the shaking to continue. Shake for as long as you feel comfortable.

- *Step 6*: Next, place your feet flat on the floor, keeping your knees slightly apart. This will allow the shaking to move into your pelvis and lower back.

Remember, shaking can be physically and emotionally tiring, and, like all exercise, shouldn't be overdone. If you start feeling tired, don't exceed 15 minutes. Similarly, if you go beyond 15 minutes, stop as soon as you feel tired.

When you're ready to stop the shaking exercise, extend your legs and place them flat onto the floor. Relax on your back or curl up on your side.

Warning – stand up slowly and carefully. Your leg and pelvic muscles will be more relaxed after shaking exercises.

Someone with PBS would be advised to carry out the exercises very carefully and gently, as, although they are releasing tension, they could bring on a flare-up, especially if someone is deficient in magnesium. There is no advantage in pushing yourself, but rather allow the process to unfold gradually over time.

You should be aware that this can be a powerful process and that strong emotions and feelings can sometimes rise to the surface. So although I have included the exercise here for information, I recommend that you only undertake it under the guidance and care of a suitably qualified practitioner. The exercises are not suitable for people with any structural problems or who suffer with back pain or have a history of whiplash or injury. Neither are they suitable for those who have a history of psychiatric illness such as schizophrenia. Your practitioner will be able to guide and support you through this process according to what you personally need.

CHAPTER 11

Acupuncture

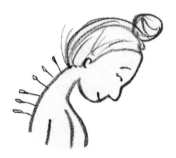

Acupuncture aims to restore equilibrium in a body which has become unbalanced by physical pain or illness or mental or emotional upset. Unlike orthodox medicine, it treats these factors as interconnected.

Acupuncturists believe that the underlying cause of pain and illness is a blockage in the flow of qi, or energy. Bad diet, injury or infection can cause this blockage, as can emotional factors. So, to get the qi moving smoothly again, acupuncturists insert fine needles into appropriate acupuncture points on the body. From the restored flow, the natural healing process can begin.

Acupuncturists focus on the patient first, the condition second – and recognise each person's symptoms as being related to one another. For this reason, two patients diagnosed with identical conditions would nevertheless be regarded as distinct cases with different needs by an acupuncturist.

Accordingly, their acupuncture treatment plan would be different too.

Acupuncture is a branch of traditional Chinese medicine. As such it has been evolving for two thousand years since the earliest known text on the subject, *The Yellow Emperor's Classic of Internal Medicine*, appeared between the first century BC and the first century AD. The origins of all styles of acupuncture practised around the world today can be found in this text. Even though the language and terminology associated with acupuncture reflect Chinese medicine's cultural and historic origins, its proponents and practitioners are every bit as scientific or sophisticated as their counterparts in orthodox western medicine in their knowledge and understanding of the human body.

Acupuncture has been shown to be more effective in relieving symptoms of PBS than strategies applied by traditional medicine. This is because research has shown that it can alleviate the emotional distress experienced by patients as well as the physical symptoms of pain, frequency and urgency. In one study, 75 per cent of respondents reported improvements in their emotional states after acupuncture treatment.

Other studies have found that:

- people with PBS can feel better after as few as ten acupuncture sessions

- pain of PBS can reduce after six to eight weeks of acupuncture.

In a Norwegian study,[65] 67 adult women with recurrent urinary tract infections (UTIs) were split into three randomised groups. The first group received acupuncture treatment; the second had pretend acupuncture; while the third group received no treatment at all. Significantly, 85 per cent of the acupuncture group was free of cystitis during the six-month observational period. This compares with 58 per cent in the sham group and only 36 per cent in the control group.

Concluding her investigation into the treatment of interstitial cystitis with acupuncture, Toni Tucker, a practitioner of traditional Chinese acupuncture, wrote:

> This study indicates that if a practitioner has a clear understanding of IC and gives suitable lifestyle advice, acupuncture can be more effective than Western medicine in the treatment of IC. Acupuncture is successful not only in treating the physical symptoms of IC, but also at improving the patient's emotional state.[66]

Fran, age 39

Fran can trace her PBS back to her first pregnancy. Her baby died in the womb and she had to deliver him stillborn. Although she fell pregnant soon after and happily gave birth to a healthy baby girl, Fran decided that she didn't want any more children and had a coil fitted.

Before long, Fran experienced heavy bleeding and, during her periods, irritation and a bearing-down sensation on her bladder. Her urethra would frequently feel hot after heavy bleeding and she had regular episodes of cystitis symptoms – which meant regular courses of antibiotics. After six months of repeated pain and infection, Fran had the coil removed.

This didn't stop the discomfort, however, and Fran continued to experience intense pain in her bladder. She had several examinations, including a cystoscopy which revealed that there was, in fact, no infection. PBS was diagnosed.

Fran decided to give acupuncture a try and is really pleased with the results. In fact, she finds it so effective that she has a session a week before her period, which results in her feeling no pain whatsoever.

CHAPTER 12

Adaptogens

Adaptogens are natural substances, found in many herbs. As their name suggests, they keep the body adaptable in the face of a wide range of pressures, most notably stress. They can also help to restore balance and maintain a healthy metabolism.

The exact benefit of adaptogens and quite what they do is difficult to pin down as, unlike many other nutrients, supplements or forms of therapy, their role is not specific to a particular function (e.g. breaking down fats or boosting white blood cells). Nor do they target specific organs in the body. Instead, the effects of adaptogens are felt in the form of a general increased vitality and a reduced vulnerability to stress.

The inherent vagueness of the role of these highly effective substances has preoccupied doctors, herbalists and physicians since the 1940s, even though their use dates back to the ancient medicines of China and India thousands of years ago. In 1947, Dr Nikolai Lazarev, a Soviet pharmacologist exploring ways to treat stress and prevent illness through homeostasis (internal stability), offered this definition:

> Adaptogen: an agent that allows the body to counter adverse physical, chemical or biological stressors by raising non-specific resistance toward such stress, thus allowing the organism to adapt to the stressful circumstances.[67]

Some 20 years later, two of Dr Lazarev's compatriots, the holistic doctors Israel L. Brekhman and L.V. Dardymov, enlarged on his definition with:

(a) an adaptogen is almost nontoxic to the recipient;

(b) an adaptogen tends to be non-specific in its pharmacological properties and acts by increasing the resistance of the organism to a broad spectrum of adverse biological, chemical, and physical factors;

(c) an adaptogen tends to be a regulator having a normalizing effect on the various organ systems of the recipient organism.[68]

These are the nearest we have to a formal definition of an adaptogen and they form the criteria for establishing if a plant or herb has adaptogenic properties. So, to be an adaptogen, a substance must:

• not be harmful in any way or cause significant side-effects, as stated in (a) above

• build adaptive energy, ideally as a reserve form of energy for use when the body comes under pressure from stress; this is what is meant by the non-specific response in (b) above

• counter bidirectional forces on bodily functions as per (c) above; so, for example, an adaptogen should help to regulate blood pressure, whether it is too high or two low.

The single most important benefit of adaptogens is that they create a reserve of adaptive energy that all major cells in the body can access.

This means that a person whose diet is rich in adaptogens is well equipped to counter assaults though both emotional and physical assaults as they help to:

- regulate the hypothalamic-pituitary-adrenal (HPA) axis, thus boosting the adrenals and helping them produce cortisol at the optimum time of the day

- achieve homeostasis during stressful periods by enabling the body to adapt to a changing hormonal environment

- maintain the body's biorhythms and time-related cycles

- optimise the body's responses to heat, cold, noise and other external pressures

- reduce inflammation

- scavenge free radicals and reduce signs of early ageing.

Some adaptogens are also known to aid liver function, in particular liver detoxification.

Thanks to their relatively loose definition, the benefits of adaptogens are open to a wide range of interpretations. As a consequence, their use varies across global cultures and medical disciplines. In Chinese medicine, for example, adaptogens are referred to as qi tonics and are used to nourish bodily organs and increase energy reserves. In Russian medicine, as we have already seen, they are regarded as vital to increase our resistance to stress and stabilise organ function, while western medicine focuses on the capacity of adaptogens to control the hypothalamic-pituitary-adrenal (HPA) axis (see page 61). In clinical herbalism, we recognise all these benefits and use adaptogens to balance the immune systems and prevent emotional stress from making a bad condition worse. Unsurprisingly, then, adaptogens have a big role to play in the treatment of PBS.

There is no definitive list of adaptogens, as new discoveries in the adaptogenic properties of plants and herbs is, even today, an ongoing and evolving process. However, it is widely recognised that the following herbs are adaptogens and these are commonly used by herbalists to help people with PBS and other physical and stress-related conditions:

- American ginseng (Panax quinquefolius)
- Ashwaganda (Withania somnifera)
- Astragalus (Astragalus membranaceus)
- Guduchi (Tinospora cordifolia)
- Holy basil (Ocimum sanctum)
- Liquorice root (Glycyrrhiza glabra)*
- Reishi (Ganoderma lucidum)
- Schisandra (Schisandra chinensis)
- Shilajit (Asphaltum bitumen)
- Shatavari (Asparagus racemosus)
- Siberian ginseng (Eleutherococcus senticosus).

*Can cause salt retention, resulting in high blood pressure, although it is a specific for those with PBS.

Sandra, age 46

For almost ten years, Sandra had major problems: extremely painful periods, heavy bleeding, almost constant pain in her lower abdomen and severe constipation. Investigative procedures pointed to severe endometriosis, so Sandra decided to have a hysterectomy.

The operation was a success in that Sandra had no more periods, but the constant ache in her lower abdomen wouldn't go away. After further investigations revealed nothing, her gynaecologist suggested seeing a urologist to check for bladder problems.

Suspecting PBS, the urologist suggested cutting out acidic foods and other known bladder aggravants. Straight away, Sandra discovered that chocolate was a major aggravant for her and if she avoided it, the pain would recede. She had also read that cranberry juice can be helpful for the bladder, but this caused a PBS flare-up.

He initially decided to prescribe just one herb – marshmallow root. The effect was instant and Sandra stated that she no longer felt any daily pain. After taking a relatively high dosage of three mugs a day to begin with, she now has only one. However, she noticed that stress could still cause a flare-up of her symptoms. It was then that her herbalist prescribed ashwaganda to be taken with her marshmallow root. The effect wasn't instant but after a couple of months she responded well and noticed that periods of stress no longer triggered a flare-up.

CHAPTER 13

The Seven Point PBS Protocol

Your Road to Recovery

When I treat patients for PBS at my clinic, I take them through a seven stage protocol. Addressing all the points discussed in this book, the protocol aims to uncover and deal with all the factors that cause the symptoms of pain, frequency and urgency with natural, safe and effective methods. This is a proven protocol and one that continues to help many people live a life free from PBS.

1. **Food and drink**: Discover which foods in your diet cause the initial aggravation and contribute to your PBS symptoms. Common aggravants are tomatoes, chocolate, coffee and alcohol. You may also be intolerant to gluten if you have PBS.

2. **Lifestyle**: Assess factors in your lifestyle that can contribute to your symptoms. These could include irregular sleeping patterns which can affect your adrenal health and cortisol production, the tightness and material of your clothes and any stress you are exposed to.

    Routine is key and creating a healthy lifestyle is fundamental to your recovery.

3. **Poisons**: Assess the level of toxins you are exposed to and their effect on your body. As well as the toxins in your home, this should include a mercury test and an evaluation of your dental condition to assess any amalgam fillings, cavitations and any obstacles to cranial motion.

   If you do have mercury fillings and decide to have then removed then it needs to be carried out by a specialist mercury-free dentist. Then, once done, you will need to carry out the mercury detox protocol (see the Appendix). Make sure there are no unresolved dental infections and that gum health is excellent.

4. **Gentle detoxification**: Experience the relaxing and cleaning effect of detoxification through skin brushing, far infrared saunas, castor oil packs and other therapies to rid your body of yeasts, mercury and other harmful toxins.

   Detoxification doesn't have to be heroic. Changing your diet, encouraging lymphatic cleansing and following the gentle liver flush (see the recipe in the Appendix) and sweating are all helpful in reducing the toxic burden in the body.

5. **Bladder and gut repair**: Re-mineralise your gut and repair the glycosaminoglycan (GAG) layer on the bladder wall with home-made bone or vegetarian broths, Epsom salt baths, herbal remedies, probiotics and dietary supplements.

   Try the bladder and restorative tea recipes and see which ones suit you (see the recipes in the Appendix).

6. **Trauma release**: Find a practitioner who can help work with you on purging your body of stored trauma, no matter how old, through somatic release such as shaking exercises. Unburden yourself of a painful past and focus on your future.

7. **Bodywork**: Complement your healing strategy with massage and/or acupuncture. If you've never had either, you'll be amazed at what they can do for you.

   Acupuncture is particularly helpful for PBS. Points that might be used are spleen 6 and Ren 3. However, I have found that in my clinic, points from the Master Tung system of acupuncture yield excellent and quick therapeutic results. Although it isn't a well-known system, it is possible to find practitioners who are able to use his system of Taiwanese acupuncture.

Conclusion

Painful bladder syndrome/interstitial cystitis is not just a disorder of the bladder. It is a condition which is related to the whole body, both in terms of the cause and its symptoms. The condition, which affects millions of people worldwide, is non-discriminating, causing untold misery for young and old, male and female.

I, as well as many other researchers into PBS, believe that the cause is usually multi-factoral. Focusing on just the bladder is not enough. The whole body has to be taken into consideration in order to stimulate the body to heal itself.

Many people turn to a holistic medical approach because of the discomfort of medical treatments or simply because they haven't worked. As I have explored through this book, I believe that natural medicine offers a very promising approach. The cause of PBS seems to vary from person to person. For one individual, mercury filling extraction offers a cessation of symptoms. For another, it is cutting out gluten or stopping the contraceptive pill.

At the hub of the seemingly unrelated symptoms and factors is the gut and digestive system. A healthy gut lining enables us to correctly process food and waste. Healthy flora protect us from toxic exposure and help us metabolise the modern onslaught of chemicals, heavy metals and drugs to which we are all exposed. Once this important gut lining becomes compromised, our immune system struggles. Toxic metabolites, never designed to get to our liver and bladder, wreak havoc. The immune system, recognising that something 'other than self' is present, attacks the tissues containing these foreign toxins. As a result, an autoimmune situation can arise. Our immune system doesn't attack itself without a reason. It is the body's attempt to deal with toxicity that has arisen as a consequence of environmental contaminants and toxins from faulty digestive processes.

Because everyone is different, it is important to find an approach which is specific to you. Individualised medicine is a necessary approach for chronic lingering disorders, and PBS is no exception.

We are not yet at a point where there has been sufficient research and trials to absolutely define the cause and treatment for PBS. The process of understanding is going to be especially cumbersome as there doesn't seem to be one single cause or therapeutic approach which clinically applies to everyone.

Although the approach which induces healing is usually eclectic, at the same time, I have found that minimal intervention is the best. People who have PBS have a situation where their body is very sensitive, whether this is to drugs, foods, supplements, herbs and so on. The immune system is on high alert as a result of toxic overload. It is imperative to keep exposure to man-made chemicals to a minimum whilst on the healing journey. This can be in the form of cleaning products, personal care products and any substance put on the skin. This also includes keeping your home environment as toxin free as possible. It might seem a bit extreme to say that you should wait for healing to take place before buying new furniture and carpets, but I have seen that a sudden exposure to, say, formaldehyde, such as in new carpets, can be enough to cause a relapse at the first stage of healing. The less your body has to detoxify the better.

The first step is finding the triggers that are affecting you; this is usually foods and drinks. Pin-pointing the foods which cause pain and discomfort is a great first step. However, this is not enough to create healing. Once that is done the restoration of a healthy balance of gut flora is paramount.

The holy grail for PBS is discovering a way to heal the GAG layer. However, in order to do this, healing needs to take place with all the mucous membranes, the most extensive one of course being the digestive system. The body will heal the GAG layer, although to do that, the constant drip of toxins attacking the lining needs to stop. Once the gut has been attended to then there are compounds which, if ingested, the body will use in GAG layer repair. Herbs are a very effective way of soothing the bladder lining and encouraging its regeneration.

Stress is a huge aggravator of PBS, slowing the healing process and disturbing the balance of hormones. So to establish healing, life changes are often needed. Ways of reducing our stress levels can seem too simple, such as eating on time and having a healthy daily routine, but I have seen that sometimes the most simple of measures can have a very important role in keeping our stress levels manageable. Because our body stores stress and emotions, as they say, 'our issues are in our tissues'. Trauma release methods as well as bodywork such as acupuncture have an enormous part to play.

The road to wellness is rarely a straight one. Setbacks can occur, and in the midst of the process it can feel overwhelming and insurmountable. It is essential to find professional therapeutic help and support, not just for your diet and healing but also for moral support and encouragement. There is always a way. This means working with your body to encourage the healing that your body is truly capable of.

APPENDIX

Recipes and Formulae

Mercury detox protocol

There are many approaches to eliminating mercury and indeed any toxic metal from the body. Not one approach will necessarily work for everyone. I strongly urge you to gain guidance from a qualified practitioner who understands how to eliminate metals in someone who has PBS. Typically I find it important for someone's symptoms to be reasonably under control before having their mercury fillings removed.

Most people can tolerate marshmallow root tea and it has a key role in supporting the mucous membrane (GAG layer) whilst you are mobilising the mercury out of your body.

As I have stressed, it is imperative that you have a dentist who is totally familiar with amalgam removal. They need to be meticulous in the extraction, and usually it needs to be done gradually.

Any heavy metal detoxification should only be undertaken once the amalgam has been removed from the teeth. Mobilising mercury out of the tissues in the body when amalgams are present in the teeth can result in increased mercury toxicity.

There are many approaches to cleaning mercury from the body. The bowel cleanse formula is particularly useful for mopping up metal residues present in the gut immediately after extraction. It is usually taken for a period of at least ten days after having your mercury fillings removed.

Bowel cleanse formula

Bowel cleanse powder is made from equal parts of the following:

- bentonite clay

- psyllium husks

- activated charcoal

- apple fruit pectin

- slippery elm inner bark.

I use a formula based on all these five ingredients in my clinic to promote detoxification of chemicals, heavy metals and radioactivity. I usually prescribe at least one teaspoon of this mixture a minimum of three times daily for a period of ten days. It is vitally important that you continue to have regular bowel movements while ingesting this, in order for the toxins to get out. Drinking prune juice, or soaking a tablespoon of linseeds in water left overnight and drinking the whole mixture in the morning normally does the trick. Drinking the linseed mixture is very helpful for chronic constipation. Herbal laxatives containing senna pods or cascara sagrada should only be used in an emergency and for a maximum of a couple of weeks.

You should mix the bowel cleanse powder in a jam jar with water or apple juice, shake it and drink it immediately. It is important to ensure that at least a litre of water is drunk throughout the day. Take it about an hour before meals, or two hours after.

One of the most remarkable plant medicines to remove heavy metals is coriander leaf (cilantro). If you can tolerate it without creating any bladder pain, then it can be added into your food and it can be taken as a herbal extract. It needs to be organic as it can be heavily sprayed.

I have found that the following formula, which is a variation of the original by the famous American herbalist Dr John Christopher, to be particularly effective.

Toxic metal detoxification formula
This formula comprises equal parts of:

- bugleweed (Lycopus virginicus)
- yellow dock (Rumex crispus)
- burdock (Arctium lappa)
- lobelia (Lobelia inflata).

For PBS patients, this formula is usually prescribed in capsule form, as herbal tinctures (which contain alcohol) can be aggravating. This formula is only available from a herbalist, as it contains the 'practitioner only' ingredient Lobelia. It is usually taken for four weeks followed by a break of two weeks before repeating. The herbalist prescribing this formula will decide the dosage, which for adults is usually 30 drops three times daily, in water before food.

After the mercury amalgam has been removed from the teeth, it can take at least 12 months for the deposits of mercury present in fat, muscle and nervous system to be excreted. However, some patients with PBS who have a mercury toxicity problem notice an improvement in their symptoms very rapidly after mercury filling extraction.

Gut balance and metal detoxification
Once the amalgam has been removed, focus should be on restoring gut bacterial balance and repairing the leaky gut. This is an absolute priority, as the body's ability to

excrete heavy metals relies on healthy bowel flora. I usually recommend that this be attended to first, and once this has been done then gentle chelation can be carried out.

People who are already weak and suffering from many symptoms should attempt to restore their gut function before attempting any kind of metal detoxification.

WARNING

People with neurological conditions such as Parkinson's disease and multiple sclerosis have extremely compromised detoxification pathways. Therefore, detoxification can be contraindicated. If cleansing is deemed suitable it should only be undertaken with the utmost care and under experienced supervision.

The liver flush

- 250ml organic cartoned or bottled pear juice

- 250ml filtered water

- 1 whole organic/unwaxed lemon (peeled leaving pith)

- 1 tbsp organic virgin olive oil

- ½ tsp turmeric powder

- a chunk of fresh ginger root about the size of your little toe

Blend all of the ingredients in a liquidiser and drink in the morning. The flush should be made fresh each time and consumed as soon as it is made. Once drunk you need to follow it with hot ginger or peppermint tea. Do not eat for at least 30 minutes after the liver flush.

Gradually increase the strength of the liver flush each day by adding one tablespoon of olive oil, up to a maximum of four tablespoons of olive oil. Maintain this level until you have finished the flush. Should this make you feel nauseous, reduce the amount of oil and try increasing in more gradual increments.

The liver flush encourages toxins to be released into the small intestine via the bile duct. For this reason, it is important that the bowels are moving regularly, providing a clear exit from the body. When we are producing and releasing the correct amount of bile, digestion is effective without leaving us feeling tired after eating. The liver flush is also very useful for treating constipation caused by a lack of bile and digestive juices. I recommend that the flush is taken every day for a minimum of one week, but for maximum medicinal benefit it should be taken daily for four weeks.

How the liver flush works

The liver flush increases the flow of bile from the liver and gall bladder, allowing the body to dump toxins from the liver into the digestive tract, for eventual elimination via the gut. Each ingredient has a favourable influence on the liver function.

- *Pear juice*: this is high in malic acid, which can render toxic metals inert and increase cellular energy. Pear juice also improves the taste of the liver flush.

- *Olive oil*: a sudden quantity of oil through the feedback mechanism in the gut stimulates large amounts of bile to pass into the small intestine.

- *Lemon*: being sour, lemon activates bile flow and the production of digestive enzymes. It also helps the digestion of the oil and makes the flush palatable.

- *Ginger*: this helps to settle the stomach and prevents nausea through the stimulation of digestive juices.

Ginger contains gingerol, a chemical that is known to counteract liver toxicity by stimulating bile excretion. It increases the level of the antioxidant enzyme, superoxide dismutase, which protects against oxidative stress.

- *Turmeric*: turmeric is an incredibly powerful detoxifier and probably the most powerful anti-inflammatory agent in nature.

The liver flush is contraindicated when there are gallstones present and should only be undertaken under the guidance of a health professional.

Herbal teas to rebuild the GAG layer

As I have mentioned, there are a number of ways to encourage the body to regenerate and repair the GAG layer. Not every approach will work for everyone, although I have found that marshmallow root (Althea officinalis) is almost always well tolerated and incredibly useful. I usually prescribe it in tea, as opposed to capsules and tincture form.

Marshmallow tea

As a basic herbal infusion, I recommend that at least 500ml is drunk daily. You can start gradually and take one cup a day to see how you respond, and bit by bit increase up to one litre of tea daily.

The marshmallow roots should be organic and correctly dried to ensure there is no mould present.

To make one litre of marshmallow tea, you will need two tablespoons of the dried root. The concentration can be increased, such as adding three tablespoons, but I haven't found it particularly more effective. Marshmallow has demulcent qualities, meaning that it contains active constituents that have a soothing and rebuilding effect on mucous membranes.

Bladder lining repair tea

This is a more complex formula which I use to encourage the repair and rebuilding of the GAG layer.

- 5 parts marshmallow root (Althea officinalis)

- 2 parts fennel seeds (Foeniculum vulgare)

- 2 parts lotus seeds (Nelumo nucifera semen; if available)

- 1 part liquorice root (Glycyrrhiza glabra radix; to be avoided in high blood pressure)

An alternative bladder lining repair tea

This formula contains ingredients that are more difficult to source and contain many ayurvedic herbs. The advanced formula is usually taken as an alternative to the previous formula.

Equal parts of:

- gokshura (Tribulas terrestris semen)

- varuna (Crataeva nurvula)

- purnanva/Indian hogweed (Boerhaavia diffusa radix)

- marshmallow root (Althea officinalis)

Either of the herbal teas should be taken (if well tolerated) every day for at least a period of a couple of months. They are more effective if at the same time bone broth is consumed. Vegetarians should take glucosamine tablets to help the repair of the GAG layer.

Broth recipes

Bone broth

- Bones: organic chicken is an absolute must. The whole chicken carcass can be used. Meat left on the bones can be added and will produce a stronger tasting stock.

- 2 tsp salt (approx.)

- ½ a lemon (this helps to break down the bones to extract the minerals and cartilage)

- Vegetables that are well tolerated can be chopped up and added, such as carrots and celery. If you can tolerate onions these can be put into the mix as well.

- Seasoning: optional, but use seasoning that you know you are okay with. In the early stages you might not be able to put any into the stock. Many PBS suffers find that parsley, thyme, rosemary, oregano and bay leaves are okay, but you have to discover what is suitable for you.

Place the bones, or in the case of a chicken, the carcass, into a large pan and cover with filtered water. Add the salt and bring it to a boil. Then add the lemon, vegetables and chosen seasoning. Cooking time varies, but at least keep it on a low simmer overnight. If time permits, 24 to 48 hours is even better; you will have to keep monitoring it to make sure it is topped with water.

It is usually better to use a slow cooker so that you can safely leave it overnight to cook.

Once you have left it for sufficient time to cook, let it cool a bit before pouring into glass jars to be stored. The mixture when cooled will usually become semi-solid, so it is better to pour into the glass containers before it has solidified. If you store it in the fridge it will last for three to five days. It can then be scooped into whichever preparation you are cooking. Examples would be stir fries, soups, casseroles and gravy. It can be frozen and you can divide it into small containers, store those in the freezer and then add into meals as and when you need. Some people put the broth into ice cube trays so they have their own ready-made medicinal stock in a convenient form.

Bone broth is usually well tolerated. However, in the rare instance it causes a flare-up or bladder discomfort you will need to reduce the amount you are taking till you can find a daily amount you can tolerate. Once this has been established you can then gradually build up the quantity day by day. You could start with a couple of tablespoons in a meal a day and then build up to consuming at least a cup of the bone broth a day.

Vegetarian mineral broth

This is a reasonable alternative to the bone broth for vegetarians. Like the bone broth, this contains minerals which are vital for repairing the GAG layer. This is a variation of the one featured in my book *Make Yourself Better*.[25]

The measurements are very approximate to give you an idea of the proportions needed.

- 100g potato peelings

- 100g carrot peelings and whole chopped beetroots

- 100g onions and garlic (this is optional, and depends on you tolerating them)

- 100g celery, dark greens and broccoli stalks

- 50g shitake mushrooms

- 2 glucosamine sulphate 500gm tablets

- shells of two eggs (if you eat eggs)

- ½ a lemon

- seasoning: optional, but use seasoning that you know you are okay with. In the early stages you might not be able to put any into the stock. Many PBS suffers find that parsley, thyme, rosemary, oregano and bay leaves are okay, but you have to discover what is suitable for you.

Place the ingredients in a large pot and cover with water. Simmer on a very low temperature for three hours. Once cooked it needs to be poured through a muslin cloth and strained. It can then be refrigerated and kept in the fridge for up to three days or frozen. It can be used as directed for bone broth.

Ghee recipe[69]
Place 2 lb of unsalted, organic butter into a heavy bottomed, stainless steel saucepan and slowly melt on a low heat.

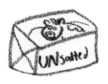 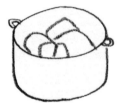

Continue to cook slowly, keeping a wary eye all the while as it burns easily if heated too fast or on too high a heat. Bubbles will be seen rising to the surface and a residue of milk solids will be seen forming on the surface. This usually clears in the middle allowing you to observe the liquid changing colour beneath and milk solids forming on the base of the pan.

When ready (about 30 mins), the ghee turns a transparent golden brown colour and bubbles begin to stop rising to the surface (the bubbles are the water content of the butter evaporating). The ghee burns very quickly at this stage so remove from the heat as soon as the milk solids on the bottom of the pan begin to turn brown and most of the bubbles have stopped rising.

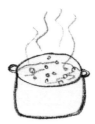

Wait until the ghee has cooled but is still in a liquid form and then strain it through a piece of muslin cloth into a suitable container – jam jars work well.

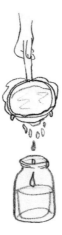

Ghee has a long shelf life if stored in tightly sealed jars. Refrigeration is unnecessary.

Endnotes

1   Homma, Y., Ueda, T., Tomoe, H., Lin, A.T.L. *et al.* (2009) 'Clinical guidelines for interstitial cystitis and hypersensitive bladder syndrome.' *International Journal of Urology 16*, 7, p.599.

2   Hurst, R.E. (2003) 'A deficit of proteoglycans on the bladder uroepithelium in interstitial cystitis.' *European Urology Supplements 2*, 4, 10–13.

3   Nickel, J.C. and Cornish, J. (1994) 'Ultrastructural study of an antibody-stabilized bladder surface: a new perspective on the elusive glycosaminoglycan layer.' *World Journal of Urology 12*, 1, 11–14.

4   www.nhs.uk/Conditions/Cystitis/Pages/Complications.aspx, accessed on 10 August 2012.

5   www.health.harvard.edu/fhg/updates/update0104d.shtml, accessed on 10 August 2012.

6   Efros, M., Bromberg, W., Cossu, L., Nakeleski, E. and Katz, A.E. (2010) 'Novel concentrated cranberry liquid blend, UTI-STAT with Proantinox, might help prevent recurrent urinary tract infections in women.' *Urology 76*, 4, 841–845.

7   Seshadri, P., Emerson, L. and Morales, A. (1994) 'Cimetidine in the treatment of interstitial cystitis.' *Urology 44*, 4, 614–616.

8   www.womenshealthmatters.ca/health-resources/pelvic-health/interstitial-cystitis/treatment, accessed on 10 August 2012.

9   www.orthoelmiron.com, accessed on 10 August 2012.

10   Edwards, T. (2005) 'Inflammation, pain, and chronic disease: an integrative approach to treatment and prevention.' *Alternative Therapies in Health and Medicine 11*, 6, 20–27; quiz 28, 75.

11   Weinstock, L., Klutke, C. and Lin, H. (2008) 'Small intestinal bacterial overgrowth in patients with interstitial cystitis and gastrointestinal symptoms.' *Digestive Diseases and Sciences 53*, 5, 1246–1251.

12   Furness, J.B., Kunze, W.A. and Clerc, N. (1999) 'Nutrient tasting and signaling mechanisms in the gut. II. The intestine as a sensory organ: neural, endocrine, and immune responses.' *American Journal of Physiology 277*, 5 Pt 1, G922–928.

13   Hill, D.A. and Artis, D. (2009) 'Intestinal bacteria and the regulation of immune cell homeostasis.' *Annual Review of Immunology 28*, 623–667.

14   Berer, K. and Krishnamoorthy, G. (2012) 'Commensal gut flora and brain autoimmunity: a love or hate affair?' *Acta Neuropathologica 123*, 5, 639–651.

15   Grölund, M.-M., Lehtonen, O.-P., Eerola, E. *et al.* (1999) 'Fecal microflora in healthy infants born by different methods of delivery: permanent changes in intestinal flora after cesarean delivery.' *Journal of Pediatric Gastroenterology and Nutrition 28*, 19–25.

16   Saarinen, U.M. and Kajosaari, M. (1995) 'Breastfeeding as prophylaxis against atopic disease: prospective follow-up study until 17 years old.' *The Lancet 346*, 8982, 1065–1069.

17   Mette, C., Tollånes, D.M, Daltveit, A.K. and Irgens, L.M. (2008) 'Cesarean section and risk of severe childhood asthma: a population-based cohort study.' *Journal of Pediatrics 153*, 1, 112–116.

18   Mei, J., Liu, Y., Dai, N., Hoffmann, C. *et al.* (2012) 'Cxcr2 and Cxcl5 regulate the IL-17/G-CSF axis and neutrophil homeostasis in mice.' *Journal of Clinical Investigation 122*, 3, 974–986. doi: 10.1172/JCI60588.

19   Zamfir, M., Callewaert, R., Cornea, P.C. and De Vuyst, L. (2000) 'Production kinetics of acidophilin 801, a bacteriocin produced by Lactobacillus acidophilus IBB 801.FEMS.' *Microbiology Letters 190*, 2, 305–308.

20   Williams, L.L. (2011) *Radical Medicine*. Vermont: Healing Arts Press.

21   Wang, F., Zhang, P., Jiang, H. and Cheng, S. (2012) 'Gut Bacterial Translocation Contributes to Microinflammation in Experimental Uremia.' *Digestive Diseases and Sciences* [Epub. ahead of print.]

22   Liu, Z., Li, N. and Neu, J. (2005) 'Tight junctions, leaky intestines, and pediatric diseases.' *Acta Paediatrica 94*, 4, 386–393.

23   Pant, C., Madonia, P. and Minocha, A. (2009) 'Does PPI therapy predispose to Clostridium difficile infection?' *Nature Reviews Gastroenterology and Hepatology 6*, 555–557.

24   Truss, C.O. (1984) 'Metabolic abnormalities in patients with chronic candidiasis: the acetaldehyde hypothesis.' *Journal of Orthomolecular Psychiatry 13*, 2, 66–93.

25   Weeks, P. (2012) *Make Yourself Better*. London: Singing Dragon.

26   Pacholok, S.M. and Stuart, J.J. (2005) *Could It Be B12?* California: Quill Driver Books.

27   Rashid, H.H., Reeder, J.E., O'Connell, M.J., Zhang, C.-O., Messing, E.M. and Keay, S.K. (2004) 'Interstitial cystitis antiproliferative factor (APF) as a cell-cycle modulator BMC.' *Urology 4*, 3.

28   Smith, L.L. (2003) 'Another cholesterol hypothesis: cholesterol as antioxidant.' *Free Radical Biology and Medicine 11*, 1, 47–61.

29   Ravnskov, U. (2004) 'High cholesterol may protect against infections and atherosclerosism.' *Quarterly Journal of Medicine 96*, 12, 927–934.

30   Gertler, M.M., Garn, S.M. and Lerman, J. (1950) 'The interrelationships of serum cholesterol, cholesterol esters and phospholipids in health and in coronary artery disease.' *Circulation 2*, 205–214.

31   Ravnskov, U. (1992) 'Cholesterol lowering trials in coronary heart disease: frequency of citation and outcome.' *British Medical Journal 305*, 6844, p.15.

32   Kunugi, H. (2001) 'Low serum cholesterol and suicidal behavior.' *Nihon Rinsho 59*, 8, p.1599.

33   Nielsen, M.L., Pareek, M. and Henriksen, J.E. (2011) 'Reduced synthesis of coenzyme Q10 may cause statin related myopathy.' *Ugeskr Laeger 173*, 46, 2943–2948.

34   Sorwell, K.G., Garten, J., Renner, L., Weiss, A. *et al.* (2012) 'Hormone supplementation during aging: how much and when?' *Rejuvenation Research 15*, 2, 128–131.

35   Hyman, M. (2004) 'The impact of mercury on human health and the environment.' *Alternative Therapies 10*, 6.

36   Water UK (2001) *Mercury Briefing Paper*. London: Water UK.

37 World Health Organization (2007) *Preventing Disease Through Healthy Environments. Exposure To Mercury: A Major Public Health Concern.* Geneva: WHO Document Production Services.

38 Biolab Medical Unit (2011) *Mercury Data Sheet.* London: Biolab Medical Unit.

39 Wojcik, D.P., Godfrey, M.E., Christie, D. and Haley, B.E. (2006) 'Mercury toxicity presenting as chronic fatigue, memory impairment and depression: diagnosis, treatment, susceptibility, and outcomes in a New Zealand general practice setting (1994–2006).' *Neuroendocrinology Letters 27*, 4, 415–423.

40 Donma, O. and Donma, M.M. (2002) 'Association of headaches and the metals.' *Biological Trace Element Research 90*, 1–3, 1–14.

41 Wojcik, D.P., Godfrey, M.E., Christie, D. and Haley, B.E. (2006) 'Mercury toxicity presenting as chronic fatigue, memory impairment and depression: diagnosis, treatment, susceptibility, and outcomes in a New Zealand general practice setting (1994–2006).' *Neuroendocrinology Letters 27*, 4, 415–423.

42 Mutter, J., Naumann, J., Walach, H. and Daschner, F. (2005) 'Amalgam risk assessment with coverage of references up to 2005.' *Gesundheitswesen 67*, 3, 204–216.

43 Cheuk, D.K. and Wong, V. (2006) 'Attention-deficit hyperactivity disorder and blood mercury level: a case-control study in Chinese children.' *Neuropediatrics 37*, 4, 234–240.

44 Schiraldi, M. and Monestier, M. (2009) 'How can a chemical element elicit complex immunopathology? Lessons from mercury-induced autoimmunity.' *Trends in Immunology 30*, 10, 502–509.

45 Störtebecker, P. (1989) 'Mercury poisoning from dental amalgam through a direct nose-brain transport.' *The Lancet 333*, 8648, 1207.

46 International Programme on Chemical Safety (1991) *Inorganic Mercury* (Environmental Health Criteria 118). Geneva: World Health Organization.

47 Palkovicova, L., Ursinyova, M., Masanova, V., Yu, Z. and Hertz-Picciotto, I. (2008) 'Maternal amalgam dental fillings as the source of mercury exposure in developing fetus and newborn.' *Journal of Exposure Science and Environmental Epidemiology 18*, 3, 326–331.

48 Health Protection Agency (n.d.) *HPA Compendium of Chemical Hazards.* Available at www.hpa.org.uk/webc/HPAwebFile/HPAweb_C/1194947406874, accessed on 10 August 2012.

49 Mutter, J., Naumann, J., Walach, H. and Daschner, F. (2005) 'Amalgam risk assessment with coverage of references up to 2005.' *Gesundheitswesen 67*, 3, p.204.

50 Hilt, B., Svendsen, K., Syversen, T., Aas, O. *et al.* (2009) 'Occurrence of cognitive symptoms in dental assistants with previous occupational exposure to metallic mercury.' *Neurotoxicology 30*, 1202–1206.

51 Samir, A.M. and Aref, W.M. (2011) 'Impact of occupational exposure to elemental mercury on some antioxidative enzymes among dental staff.' *Toxicology and Industrial Health 27*, 9, 779–786.

52 Moen, B., Hollund, B. and Riise, T.J. (2008) 'Neurological symptoms among dental assistants: a cross-sectional study.' *Journal of Occupational Medicine and Toxicology 18*, 3, 10.

53 Chaitow, L. (2005) *Cranial Manipulation: Theory and Practice.* Oxford: Elsevier Churchill Livingstone.

54 Cohen, W. (2011) *The Better Bladder Book.* Alameda, CA: Hunter House.

55 Schaeffer, A.J., Amundsen, S.K. and Jones, J.M. (1980) 'Effect of carbohydrates on adherence of Escherichia coli to human urinary tract epithelial cells.' *Infection and Immunology 30*, 2, 531–537.

56 Hudson, T. (2008) *Women's Encyclopedia of Natural Medicine*. New York: McGraw Hill.

57 Korting, G.E., Smith, S.D., Wheeler, M.A., Weiss, R.M. and Foster, H.E. Jr. (1999) 'A randomized double-blind trial of oral L-arginine for treatment of interstitial cystitis.' *Journal of Urology 161*, 2, 558–565.

58 Katske, F., Shoskes, D.A., Sender, M., Poliakin, R., Gagliano, K. and Rajfer, J. (2001) 'Treatment of interstitial cystitis with a quercetin supplement.' *Techniques in Urology 7*, 1, 44–46.

59 Jernberg, C., Löfmark, S., Edlund, C. and Jansson, J.K. (2010) 'Long-term impacts of antibiotic exposure on the human intestinal microbiota.' *Microbiology 156*, 11, 3216–3223.

60 Ho, P.L., Wong, R.C., Lo, S.W., Chow, K.H., Wong, S.S. and Que, T.L. (2010) 'Genetic identity of aminoglycoside-resistance genes in Escherichia coli isolates from human and animal sources.' *Journal of Medical Microbiology 59*, 6, 702–707.

61 Campbell-McBride, N. (2010) *Gut and Psychology Syndrome*. Cambridge: Mediform UK.

62 Krohn, J. and Taylor, F. (2000) *Natural Detoxification* (2nd edition). Vancouver, BC: Hartley & Marks, p.7.

63 Stanford, E. and McMurphy, C. (2007) 'There is a low incidence of recurrent bacteria in painful bladder syndrome/interstitial cystitis patients followed longitudinally.' *International Urogynecology Journal 18*, 5, 551–554.

64 Berceli, D. (2008) *The Revolutionary Trauma Release Process: Transcend Your Toughest Times*. Vancouver: Namaste.

65 Aune, A., Alraek, T., LiHua, H. and Baerheim, A. (1998) 'Acupuncture in the prophylaxis of recurrent lower urinary tract infection in adult women.' *Scandinavian Journal of Primary Health Care 16*, 1, 37–39.

66 Holford, E. and Tucker, T. (2010) 'An investigation into the treatment of interstitial cystitis with acupuncture.' *Journal of Chinese Medicine 94*, p.31.

67 Winston, D. (2007) *Adaptogens*. Rochester, Vermont: Healing Arts Press, p.17.

68 Brekhman. I.I. and Dardymov, I.V. (1969) 'New substances of plant origin which increase nonspecific resistance.' *Annual Review of Pharmacology 9*, 419–430.

69 Cavanagh, D. and Willis, C. (2004) *The Practical Guide to Healthy Living*. Burton on Trent: Ayurveda Services Limited, p.163.

Bibliography

Alexander, K. (2007) *Dietary Healing.* Belair, South Australia: Annexus Pty Ltd.

Bartram, T. (1995) *Encyclopaedia of Herbal Medicine.* Christchurch, Dorset: Grace Publishers.

Brady, D. (2009) *IC Naturally.* Bloomington, IN: Xlibris Corporation.

Brizman, M. (2007) 'Treating interstitial cystitis with an integrative model of classical Chinese and western medicines.' Dissertation for the American University of Complementary Medicine.

Campbell-McBride, N. (2010) *Gut and Psychology Syndrome.* Cambridge: Mediform UK.

Campion, K. (1995) *The Family Medical Herbal.* London: Leopard Books.

Chaitow, L. (2005) *Cranial Manipulation.* London: Elsevier.

Cohen, W. (2011) *The Better Bladder Book.* Alameda, CA: Hunter House.

Holford, P. (2004) *The New Optimum Nutrition Bible.* London: Piatkus.

Hudson, T. (2008) *Women's Encyclopaedia of Natural Medicine.* New York: McGraw Hill.

Kilmartin, A. (2002) *The Patient's Encyclopaedia of Cystitis, Sexual Cystitis, Interstitial Cystitis.* Ohio: Bookmasters inc.

Kirkman, M. F. (2002) *The Digestive Contract, Intestinal Microbiology and Probiotics.* Kent: Biopathica Ltd.

Krohn, J. and Taylor, F. (2000) *Natural Detoxification.* Vancouver: Hartley & Marks.

Lipski, E. (2004) *Digestive Wellness.* New York: McGraw Hill.

Macallan, S. (1999) *The Mercury Papers.* Available at www.stephenmacallan.co.uk/the_mercury_papers.htm, accessed on 29 November 2011.

Montignac, M. (2010) *Glycemic Index Diet.* Monaco: Alpen Editions.

Pacholok, S. M. and Stuart, J. J. (2005) *Could it be B12? An Epidemic of Misdiagnoses.* Fresno, CA: Quill Driver Books.

Pitchford, P. (2002) *Healing with Whole Foods: Asian Traditions and Modern Nutrition.* Berkeley, CA: North Atlantic Books.

Pole, S. (2013) *Ayurvedic Medicine.* London: Singing Dragon.

Schimmel, H.W. (1997) *Functional Medicine.* Heidelberg: Haug.

Simone, C. M. (2000) *Along the Healing Path.* Ohio: IC Hope Ltd.

Simone, C. M. (2011) *IC Hope* – DVD. Ohio: IC Hope Ltd.

Turner, R. (1990) *Naturopathic Medicine.* Wellingborough: Thorsons.

Vogel, A. (1990) *The Nature Doctor.* Edinburgh: Mainstream Publishing.

Weeks, P. (2012) *Make Yourself Better.* London: Singing Dragon.

Winston, D. (2007) *Adaptogens.* Rochester, Vermont: Healing Arts Press.

Williams, L. L. (2011) *Radical Medicine.* Vermont: Healing Arts Press.

Willis, A. K. (2003) *Solving the Interstitial Cystitis Puzzle.* Los Angeles, LA: Holistic Life Enterprises.

Resources

Association of Master Herbalists
Herbalists trained in the tradition of Dr John Christopher and Richard Schulze.
www.associationofmasterherbalists.co.uk

Biolab Medical Unit
One of the laboratories that I use to assess vitamin and mineral profiles, including red cell magnesium, which also provides gut permeability testing and dysbiosis. To access tests you will need a referral from a qualified practitioner.
www.biolab.co.uk

College of Integrated Chinese Medicine
Acupuncture training college based in Reading, which teaches an integrated approach of Traditional Chinese Medicine (TCM) and 5 Element Acupuncture.
www.acupuncturecollege.org.uk

Helios Homeopathic Pharmacy
Manufacture and sell a huge range of homeopathic medicines.
www.helios.co.uk

The Nutri Centre
A huge range of supplements and remedies and an extensive health and personal development bookshop.
www.nutricentre.com

Philip Weeks Clinic
The author's clinic, providing personal consultations, individualised assessments and testing, probiotics and herbal teas.
www.philipweeks.co.uk

Wholistic Research Company
Suppliers of juicers, rebounders, enema kits, and so on.
www.wholisticresearch.com

Index